FORENSIC TOXICOLOGY

Medico-Legal Case Studies

Kalipatnapu N. Rao

CRC Press
Taylor & Francis Group
Boca Raton London New York

CRC Press is an imprint of the
Taylor & Francis Group, an **informa** business

CRC Press
Taylor & Francis Group
6000 Broken Sound Parkway NW, Suite 300
Boca Raton, FL 33487-2742

First issued in paperback 2020

ISBN-13: 978-1-4398-6681-8 (hbk)
ISBN-13: 978-0-367-77832-3 (pbk)

Library of Congress Cataloging-in-Publication Data

Rao, Kalipatnapu N.
    Forensic toxicology : medico-legal case studies / Kalipatnapu N. Rao.
        p. cm.
    Summary: "This book illustrates how analytical methods are set up, results are generated, and quality control is maintained in clinical toxicology laboratories. Geared to the practicing toxicologist who must be able to give a deposition and write a report for legal use, the book describes fifty case studies to show the progression of toxicology findings from the laboratory to the courtroom. Both civil and criminal cases are addressed, and interesting issues are explored, such as whether consumption of poppy seeds can result in a positive lab test for opiates"-- Provided by publisher.
    Includes bibliographical references and index.
    ISBN 978-1-4398-6681-8 (hardback)
    1. Forensic toxicology--Case studies. 2. Criminal investigation. I. Title.

RA1228.R36 2012
614'.13--dc23   2011035567

Visit the Taylor & Francis Web site at
http://www.taylorandfrancis.com

and the CRC Press Web site at
http://www.crcpress.com

This book is dedicated to my loving wife and friend,
Rama Rao

Contents

14   False-Positive Blood Alcohol   97

Preface

Pursuit of truth is pursuit of God

Mahatma Gandhi

Pursuit of science is pursuit of truth
Therefore, pursuit of science is pursuit of God

My father the late Kalipatnapu Sambasivarao, Ph.D.

Pursuit of law and justice is pursuit of truth
Therefore, pursuit of law and justice is pursuit of God

Kalipatnapu N. Rao, Ph.D.

This book is a first genuine effort to bridge the gap between the medical and legal professions. There are no other books on the market to deal with this issue. The title of this book, *Forensic Toxicology: Medico-Legal Case Studies*, very appropriately depicts the aim of this book.

The aims of the medical profession and the legal profession are not mutually exclusive. These two professions strive to ameliorate human suffering. A toxicologist is called upon to identify the toxin involved so that the patient can be treated adequately to get better. The legal profession also wants a toxicologist to identify whether a particular toxin at the presumptive dose used is responsible for the symptoms a defendant was allegedly exhibiting as signs of intoxication. Dose ingested determines the patient management protocols. Similarly, the nature of the ingested dose decides the punishment for the defendant.

Modern technology with state-of-the-art equipment can identify almost any toxin used in committing a crime. It is now possible to identify and quantify approximately 70 elements in the periodic table by inductively coupled plasma mass spectrometry (ICP-MS). Gas chromatography (GC) can now quantify most volatile compounds. Similarly combining GC with mass spectrometry (GC-MS) can now identify and quantify thousands of compounds. The resolving power of GC-MS can be improved by tandem mass spectrometry. Compounds can be seperated by high-pressure liquid chromatography (HPLC). It is now possible to identify several drugs used in therapeutic drug monitoring by combining liquid chromatography (LC) with mass spectrometry (LC-MS). The list of techniques goes on and if a method is not available, a forensic toxicologist can easily develop one.

The legal profession should know that the operations of a toxicology laboratory are very well organized so that an analysis done at two different laboratories with identical methods gives identical results. Congress enacted a law in 1988 called the Clinical Laboratory Improvement Amendment (CLIA), which established rules on laboratory operations.

The book is organized in such a way that medical and legal professions can understand the operations of hospital laboratories and the operations of the U.S. legal system.

Acknowledgments

I am greatly indebted to several individuals for their help, compassion, kindness, and patience, which shaped me as a scientist and a toxicologist. First, I need to thank Dr. D. Subrahmanyam for training me in lipids. This enabled me to move to the laboratory of Benito Lombardi, MD at the Department of Pathology, University of Pittsburgh in 1971. Dr. Lombardi has been a fatherly figure to me. As my mentor, he taught me how to think logically in designing experiments, how to write a manuscript, and how to effectively present results at scientific meetings. He has been a constant source of encouragement in writing this book. I wish to express my utmost gratitude to George Michalopoulos, MD, Ph.D., the Chairman of Pathology, for his encouragement and support during my stay in the department. I also thank my colleagues in the department and, in particular, Joseph Amenta, MD for his advice. I have learned a great deal from the technologists in the toxicology laboratory and their advice in developing the concept of this book. The advice and counsel provided by Ms. Mary Jane Horney, Supervisor, and Ms. Bonnie Beiler, lead technologist, were quite valuable, and the expert technical assistance provided by Mr. Edward P. Brady is appreciated. My special appreciation and gratitude is for Darla Lower, who managed the toxicology laboratory with professionalism and advised me during the development of this manuscript. I respectfully thank more than 100 very remarkable attorneys who showed confidence in me and gave me the opportunity to work as an expert witness in toxicology.

Librarians and the staff of Falk Library, University of Pittsburgh Medical Center, deserve my special thanks for their kindness and patience, which helped me immensely in putting together the manuscript for this book. I thank members of CRC Press/Taylor & Francis for giving me the opportunity to write this book. The kindness, compassion, and patience shown by Becky McEldowny Masterman, Senior Acquisition Editor, are responsible to a measurable extent for the book to take up a final shape. The guidance given by Amy Blalock, Senior Project Coordinator, Editorial Project Development was invaluable to me in developing the final manuscript. I would also like to thank Jay Margolis, Sophie Kirkwood, and everyone else at Taylor & Francis for the publication of this book.

I thank my son, Babu Rao and his wife, Srirukmini Rao for setting up my new computer and for all the software support; my daughters, Padma and

Uma and their respective husbands, Joseph and Raman, for the enlightened discussions; and my grandchildren, Joe Joe, Sandhya, and Radha for editorial assistance. I am also grateful to my youngest brother, Gopal Rao who came to my need whenever I wanted and was of great help in compiling the manuscript. Special mention should be made about my wife, Rama who has been a friend, companion, and advisor and who showed her unyielding love and devotion. She has helped me enormously in editing the manuscript.

Disclaimer

This book is presented solely for educational purposes. The author and publisher are not offering it as legal, accounting, or other professional services advice. While best efforts have been used in preparing this book, the author and publisher make no representations or warranties of any kind and assume no liabilities of any kind with respect to the accuracy or completeness of the contents. Neither the author nor the publisher shall be held liable or responsible to any person or entity with respect to any loss or incidental or consequential damages caused, or alleged to have been caused, directly or indirectly, by the information contained herein. Every case is different and the advice and strategies contained herein may not be suitable for your situation. The characters, places and entities are fictional. Any likeness to actual persons, either living or dead, is strictly coincidental.

The Author

Dr. Kalipatnapu N. Rao is an internationally recognized expert in the field of clinical chemistry and pathology. He retired from the University of Pittsburgh Medical Center (UPMC) in 2004 as a Professor of Pathology after 35 years of research and teaching. He currently holds an appointment of Adjunct Professor. Dr. Rao obtained his Ph.D. in chemistry in 1965 from the Indian Agricultural Research Institute, New Delhi, India.

Dr. Rao had a significant number of publications on the pathogenesis of acute hemorrhagic pancreatitis. He also published extensively on the nutritional aspects of pancreatic acinar cell carcinoma, breast cancer, and liver cancer, and established the importance of cholesterol metabolism in carcinogenesis.

As Chief of the Section of Toxicology and Therapeutic Drug Monitoring in the Division of Clinical Chemistry at UPMC, he published several papers in many areas of toxicology and showed that enzymatic methods utilizing alcohol dehydrogenase and NAD give false-positive serum alcohol levels in patients with elevated circulating lactate and lactate dehydrogenase enzyme. He also established that sequential monitoring of serum biomarkers for cell necrosis and regeneration could predict the outcome of liver necrosis.

Dr. Rao was an invited speaker at several national and international scientific meetings. After retiring from UPMC, he started a new career as an expert witness in toxicology. He testified in several courts throughout the country. His expertise and broad recognition in the field of toxicology helped both prosecution and defense lawyers. He gave several depositions, wrote several toxicology reports, and testified in several courts throughout the country. He was an invited speaker at Pennsylvania Bar Association, Workers' Compensation Section's annual meeting in 2004 in Hershey, Pennsylvania.

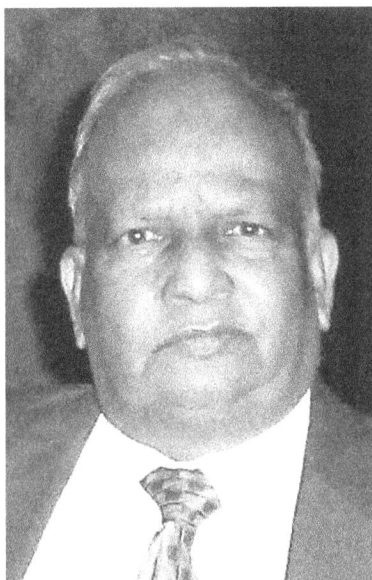

He taught first-year medical students. He trained many residents in surgery and pathology. Several undergraduate students, graduate students, and postdoctoral fellows were trained in his laboratory. He was on several Ph.D. theses advisory committees.

Historical Perspectives in Toxicology

1

1.1 Toxicology

Toxicology can be defined as a science dealing with the adverse effects of chemicals and toxins on living cells. The word toxin is derived from Greek, which means a poison. The effects on the cell are described as toxicity. The person who is knowledgeable on the effects of toxins is called a toxicologist. The recognition of toxicology as an independent science is quite recent and its evolution as a scientific discipline combining the knowledge of biology and chemistry has been quite rapid. Further impetus to this evolution is due to phenomenal developments in medicine. The discovery of new medicines to alleviate human pain and suffering necessitated the discovery of new analytical methods to monitor the drug levels in body fluids. The abuse of prescription medications requires the detection of these drugs in body fluids. Thus, the modern, clinical toxicology laboratory with state-of-the-art equipment evolved. This required moving what was once a small laboratory in a physician's office to a centralized laboratory. This development of a centralized laboratory and its organization will be discussed in detail in other chapters. Another significant development is that it required the services of a forensic toxicologist. As society evolved into organized government, well-established legislative bodies, and established judiciary and law enforcement, forensic toxicologists were required to interpret the results obtained in a central laboratory. Thus, a toxicologist evolved from a homicidal prisoner in earlier times to a scientist who helps physicians and lawyers to identify the toxin causing intoxication on their clients (1–6).

1.2 Poison

A poison was considered a coward's weapon. A poison is defined as a chemical that can sicken or kill another organism. An ideal poison is one that is effective in a very small dose and difficult to detect. As the times changed, obscure poisons were introduced. Some of them were lethal drugs like fentenyl, insulin, and muscle relaxants. Some household chemicals like antifreeze were used to commit murder for insurance money. Arsenic was a common agent to commit murder (7). With the growth of the science of clinical toxicology and forensic toxicology, the development of centralized laboratory facilities, and the availability of sophisticated analytical tools like gas chromatography (GC), gas chromatography/mass spectrometry (GC-MS), high-pressure liquid chromatography (HPLC), and liquid chromatography/ mass spectrometry (LC-MS) it became easy to detect almost any poison. With the use of an inductively coupled plasma (ICP) mass spectrometer, it is now possible to detect and quantitate up to 70 elements in the periodic table. It is also possible to extract toxin from the hair and fingernails and quantify metals, drugs, or a toxin trapped in these matrices. Today, no matter the poison, a method is easily being developed to detect it (**6**). If the present analytical methods are inadequate, forensic toxicologists develop new methods to detect and quantify any new toxin that is being used and abused.

The growth of complex centralized forensic toxicology laboratory facilities is discussed in Chapter 2.

1.3   Industrial Revolution

During the industrial revolution, there were explosive discoveries of chemicals. These chemicals are useful as well as harmful to humans. These chemicals found use as medicines and in the treatment of diseases. Discovery of pesticides enhanced food production. Introduction of plastics facilitated the storage and transport of a variety of products. The use of chemicals and the waste products released into the environment created toxic reactions in humans and animals. It was soon realized that all substances are poisons and there are none that are not poisons. The right dose distinguishes a poison from a remedy (Paracelus, 1492–1541). Industrial chemicals were found to be quite harmful when exposed in higher doses. This resulted in toxicology branching off into environmental toxicology, pharmacology, general toxicology, clinical toxicology, forensic toxicology, and occupational toxicology (**5,6**).

1.4   Effect of Insurance Industry on Homicides

The growth of the insurance industry and the ready availability of arsenic-trioxide, which is a tasteless compound without any smell, gave a stimulus to homicidal poisoning for personal gain (**7**). Even in modern times, arsenic is being used despite the fact that toxicologists can easily detect this element in body fluids of victims. It is indeed interesting to hear about homicides committed using arsenic on family members for insurance money. A forensic toxicology laboratory can easily detect arsenic in the body and aid law enforcement to bring to justice the perpetrators of these homicides.

1.5   What the Book Is About

This book is essentially about the exciting science of forensic toxicology with illustrative medico-legal case studies to show how this science acts as a bridge between medicine and law. Both of these professions strive to make the life of their clients better. The medical profession protects the physical health of a person, while the legal profession protects the freedom and well-being of a person. Chapters 2 and 3 are devoted to explaining the organization and operations involved in hospital settings. Chapters 7 and 8 are devoted to discussing the nature of several toxins with illustrative medical cases that might come to a hospital. Chapter 9 explains the nature and operations of the American legal system. Finally, legal cases illustrate how law enforcement and the court system try to protect the freedom of an individual as well as that of society as a whole.

As stated earlier, the role of a toxicologist has changed from a homicidal poisoner to an essential important scientist for medico-legal professionals. Poisons were used for centuries as a weapon of choice to commit murder. When used in the right dose, a poison can effectively kill the victim mimicking death due to natural causes. Toxicologists play an important role in detecting the cause of death. A toxicologist is called upon to determine whether a death is accidental, suicide, or homicide. In addition, forensic toxicologists play a pivotal role in determining substance abuse or an adverse reaction to a prescription medication. A toxicologist may be asked to test for carbon monoxide poisoning, or the presence of γ-hydroxy butyrate (GHB) and other date rape drugs. Society expects a toxicologist to identify environmental pollution and adverse reactions to pesticide exposure. A toxicologist is expected to identify accidental deaths secondary to the simultaneous use of alcohol and drugs such as opium, morphine, and heroin. A toxicologist is asked to identify commonly used poisons to commit crimes such as atropine, strychnine, thallium, antimony, arsenic, and cyanide (**8**).

In the emergency room, physicians are asked to find antidotes for overdose of drugs and poisons. Indeed, such antidotes are available. Tylenol overdose is treated with N-acetyl cysteine, warfarin overdose is treated with vitamin K, narcotic/opioid overdose is treated with naloxone, iron and other heavy metal overdoses are treated with deforoximine, effects of benzodiazepines are treated with flumazenil, ethylene glycol poisoning is treated with ethanol/fomepizole, and methanol poisoning is treated with ethanol or fomepizole (**6,8**).

References

1. Levine, B. *Principles of Forensic Toxicology*. AACC Press, Washington, D.C., 1999.

2. Karch, S. B. *Karch's Pathology of Drug Abuse*, 3rd ed. CRC Press, New York, 2001.
3. Burtis, C. A. and Ashwood, E. R. (Eds.) *Tietz Textbook of Clinical Chemistry*, 2nd ed. W.B. Saunders Company, Philadelphia, PA, 1994.
4. Trestrail, J. A. *Criminal Poisoning*. Humana Press, Totowa, NJ, 2000.
5. Monosson, E. History of toxicology. www.eoearth.org/article/History _of_toxi-cology.1–3, 2008.
6. Borzelica, J. The art, the science and the seduction of toxicology. An evolution-ary development. In: *Principles and Methods of Toxicology*, Hayes, A. (Ed.). Taylor & Francis, London, 2001.
7. BBC Home. A brief history of poisoning. http://www.bbc.co.uk/dna/h2g2/A4350755.
8. Ramsland, K. The first forensic science. http://trutv.com/library/crime/crimi-nal_mind/forensics/toxicology/2.html.

Organization of the Clinical Toxicology Laboratory

2

This chapter deals with the organization of the complex central clinical laboratories. It deals with the development of the concept of a central laboratory where samples are brought in from peripheral locations including physicians' offices. This resulted in cost cutting and analysis of complex tests at one location. This chapter is organized into the growth of a central laboratory, guidelines, accreditation, procedure manual writing, proficiency testing, quality control, laboratory inspections, method validation, laboratory management, and words of wisdom. The guidelines for the organization of clinical laboratories in the United States ensure uniform quality throughout the country. The reader will gain basic understanding as to what goes on when a patient's sample is tested in a laboratory.

2.1 The Growth of a Central Laboratory

In the beginning, laboratory testing was limited to few basic analytes of body fluids to aid in the diagnosis of a patient's condition by a physician. The required testing was carried out in the physician's office. Once the causative agent and etiology of diseases were understood, new diseases emerged that required new remedies. New test methods were developed to measure the newly discovered drugs and their metabolites. Some drugs were found to be toxic at higher doses. This required measuring drug levels in body fluids and establishing therapeutic windows for effective treatment. It became necessary to develop new test methods with state-of-the-art instruments, qualified technologists to conduct the testing, and experienced and qualified forensic toxicologists to manage the laboratory and to interpret the results. It became necessary to move the testing from a doctor's office to a central location. Thus, central clinical laboratories emerged. Now, a physician obtains a patient's body fluids in the office and sends them to a laboratory or sends the patient to a central laboratory where the body fluids are obtained and analyzed. Recent developments include a pneumatic tube system whereby body fluids obtained from patients on a hospital floor can be sent directly to the laboratory. The body fluids are analyzed and the results are promptly sent to the ordering physician, or put in a computer so that the ordering physician can access the results immediately.

2.2   Guidelines

The Clinical and Laboratory Standards Institute published guidelines for toxicology and drug testing in the clinical laboratory. These guidelines addressed drug testing, both for clinical and forensic purposes. These guidelines include pre-analytical, analytical, and post-analytical considerations for specimen collection, test methods, quality control, and reporting and interpretation of results (1). The number of tests performed by a clinical hospital laboratory multiplied into the thousands and became more and more complex requiring state-of-the-art equipment. The need for qualified technologists to perform these tests became obvious. The differences between clinical and forensic drug testing is recognized; however, they are not mutually exclusive. In general, requirements for forensic drug testing are quite stringent. Therefore, a hospital laboratory makes a conscious decision whether it wants to do the testing for patient care as well as for forensics. Some hospital laboratories may do both. Even when drug testing was performed for patient care only, a court may subpoena the hospital records later. Thus, any toxicology test in a clinical laboratory has the potential to become a forensic test. Differences between clinical testing and forensic testing become blurred. For an example, when a sample from a pregnant woman is positive for drugs then she could be prosecuted for fetus endangerment. Patient samples from the emergency room that test positive for drugs of abuse may have forensic implications in case of accidents that resulted in fatalities. In case of death of a patient, a coroner or a medical examiner may subpoena samples that were analyzed by the hospital toxicology laboratory, as well as the samples that were generated by a pathologist during autopsy. The results obtained by the analysis of these samples in the toxicology laboratory may have forensic implications (1).

The World Health Organization published principles and guidelines for developing medical toxicology services. These guidelines included development of an analytical toxicology laboratory. The evidence generated in a toxicology laboratory becomes important in a court of law. Acutely poisoned patients when brought to a hospital emergency room oftentimes do not require laboratory analysis. However, some patients require analysis of body fluids for analytes to monitor vital functions, as well as toxin levels. Reliable analytical methods can identify exposure to environmental poisons such as lead and mercury. Procedures must be in place for pre-analytical considerations such as appropriate sample collection and their transport to the laboratory. Analytical considerations include the use of validated, tried, and tested methods. Post-analytical considerations include interpretation of the results and their prompt communication to the clinicians. It is important that the laboratory has qualified personnel and state-of-the-art equipment to do the testing. Another essential requirement is adequate space for research and development. Depending upon the local requirements of the medical center, the laboratory may have the capacity to test for acetylcholinesterase and cholinesterase. Patients subjected to accidental chemical incidents such as massive spills and exposures as well as patients with drugs of abuse, herbal and ethnic remedies, or toxicity of drug overdoses may come to the emergency room. Patients exposed to solvents, other volatile substances, toxic alcohols such as methanol and ethylene glycols, and chlorinated and organophosphorous pesticides may also come to the hospital and the toxicology laboratory needs to be equipped to analyze these samples (2).

2.3   Accreditation

In the United States, all laboratories operate under CLIA 88 rules. Congress passed the Clinical Laboratory Improvement Amendments (CLIA) in 1988, establishing quality standards for all laboratory testing to ensure the accuracy, reliability, and timeliness of patient test results regardless of where the test was performed (3,4). All laboratories need to be certified and accredited. The qualifications and experience of personnel supervising and performing the tests are described in the Clinical Laboratory Improvement Amendment (CLIA) (3,5).

2.4   Procedure Manual

A procedure manual should be available to, and used by, the personnel at the workbench and must include principle, clinical significance, specimen type, required reagents, calibration, control procedural steps, calculations, reference ranges, and interpretation (6). A procedure manual is an important document and requires great care in its preparation. Any experienced laboratory practitioner can perform an unfamiliar procedure by looking at the procedure manual. A procedure manual, prepared for use at the workbench in the laboratory, should be explicit, unequivocal, and complete. It should be easy to follow and contain all necessary information. The guidelines require the following information for each procedure.

1. Principles and purpose of the test
2. Specimen requirements and collection method
3. Reagents, standards, controls, and matrix used
4. Instrumentation, including calibration protocols and schedules
5. Step-by-step directions, result reporting and troubleshooting, and corrective actions
6. Calculations

7. Frequency and tolerance of controls, and corrective actions to be taken if tolerances are exceeded
8. Expected values, values requiring notifications (panic/alert values), and interpretation of values
9. References
10. Effective date and schedule for review
11. Distribution
12. Author

These guidelines impose standardized structure on the quality of manuals in the laboratory (7). It is expected that there will be variations in the periodic review of the procedure manuals. It is expected that the supervising technologist sign it by putting the date on which it is reviewed. Finally, the professional staff in charge of the laboratory signs it before it is used. The supervisor corrects and signs off on any mistakes.

2.5   Proficiency Testing

The College of American Pathologists (CAP) offers proficiency testing (PT) as a part of their accreditation program. As a part of this program it offers CAP-UT (UT toxicology, which is for screening only, no confirmation), and CAP-FUDT (forensic testing, which includes screening and confirms initial testing by GC-MS). In order to be accredited, a laboratory must successfully complete a series of PT cycles for the FUDT. CAP will assemble an inspection team, which will go to the laboratory to be inspected, and review the records of prior completed PT performances. The team will assess the adequacy of the instrumentation and the qualification and training of technical staff. If deficiencies are noted, the laboratory has 30 days to correct them (6). Big laboratories participate in CAP proficiency surveys, as well as the proficiency surveys conducted by the state. For Pennsylvania, surveys require that there must be at least 15 samples per year per analyte. Pennsylvania surveys consist of blood lead, blood and/or serum alcohol, blood and/or serum drugs of abuse, and urine drugs of abuse (8). The requirements for other states may vary. Generally, there must be at least five samples per testing event. Three to four challenges a year are expected. A target value is established for each analyte, and the laboratory is expected to get a value ±10 to 25% of the target value. Here it becomes useful to add a comment regarding proficiency testing. The agencies that regulate the performance of the laboratories find proficiency testing an economical and rapid way of comparing the performance of the laboratories scattered all over the country. The laboratories also find proficiency testing is useful to compare with one another. The number of drugs used by a society is enormous, and the laboratory has to select the drugs to be analyzed depending upon its requirements. Ethanol, barbiturates, acetaminophen, and benzodiazepines are some of a few drugs that are analyzed in emergency toxicology. Opiates, amphetamines, cocaine and its metabolites, and barbiturates, etc. are usually analyzed when looking for drugs of abuse. Phenobarbital, carbamazepine, theophylline, digoxin, and gentamicin are analyzed when looking for therapeutic drugs. With the introduction of organ transplant programs, new drugs such as cyclosporine, tracolimus, and rapamycin are tested (9). Thus, a proficiency testing is done for new as well as old drugs (10-12).

2.6 Quality Control

In dealing with live biological samples, some degree of variation is expected. Because of this, quality control (QC) and quality assurance (QA) programs are introduced. CLIA 88 rules mandate that clinical laboratories put in place QC programs in conducting test procedures. Simple tests are exempt from CLIA 88 requirements; moderate and highly complex tests are subject to guidelines that include minimum personnel qualifications and laboratory proficiency tests, as well as methods and equipment to ensure proper test performance and accurate results. These guidelines for QC are intended for reliable test results and patient safety. For each test system, the laboratory is responsible for conducting the process with accuracy and precision. The QC process should be able to detect immediately the errors and monitor the test every day. The test controls should be treated in the same manner as the patient samples. The controls should be obtained from a different source other than the manufacturer, who made the reagents for any given test process (13). In the clinical laboratory, QC and QA are designed to test the performance of a procedure. The performance of the controls is plotted on a chart to compare the observed value over the expected mean over a period. These charts are called Levey-Jennings plots, and they provide visual display of method performance (14). In general, calibrators are run with every lot of new reagents or at least every 6 months. The controls are used in every run, and consist of a negative and two levels of positive controls. The QC charts are reviewed by the lead technologist daily, and reviewed by the toxicologist in charge every month. These QC records are stored in the toxicology laboratory for at least two years.

2.7 Laboratory Inspections

CAP inspects the laboratory at periodic intervals using qualified inspectors. CAP gathers qualified inspectors from equivalent sister institutions. CAP makes use of laboratory personnel who are currently active in the field. It is expected that the lab participate in proficiency testing of all analytes. The inspectors use standard checklists to carry out the inspections. The CAP checklists cover all aspects of laboratory functions. At present, there are about 18 checklists and 3200 questions. These checklists are updated regularly. Every laboratory gets a laboratory checklist and a team leader's checklist. If deficiencies are noted, they are grouped as Phase I and Phase II deficiencies. Phase I deficiencies must be corrected but require no documented response to CAP. Phase II deficiencies require documentation in responding to CAP. Laboratories have 30 days to correct the deficiencies. Sometimes, the CAP inspectors make recommendations and these do not need a response (8-11). The laboratory is mandated to maintain QA and QC programs necessary and appropriate for the validity and reliability of the test results generated for all tests performed. It should maintain procedure manuals, proper records, equipment, and facilities necessary for the proper and effective operation of the laboratory. It is mandated to participate in an approved proficiency-testing program (5). CAP, which carries out laboratory accreditation in the United States, uses the guidelines published by the National Committee for Clinical Laboratory Standards (NCCLS) (6). CAP inspectors perform laboratory inspections once every two years. The laboratory supervisors or the residents of pathology, using CAP checklists, perform the internal inspections in the years in which the inspections by CAP are not done.

2.8 Validation of New Methods

The introduction of a new instrument, a new set of reagents for new methods, or the evaluation of new reagents for a revised method is a recurring and ongoing task in every laboratory. When selecting a new method or an instrument, consideration is given to the type of specimens, sample size, throughput, specimen handling, run size, personnel skill needed, cost per test, method of calibration, capability of random access, space needed for reagent storage, and waste disposal requirements (15). It is important that the laboratory tests used are accurate and the methods employed are reliable. Otherwise, the data obtained may be contested in court, may lead to unforeseen legal consequences for the defendant, and may affect patient care. Therefore, the laboratory is expected to use accurate methods as well as reliable instrumentation. For this reason, new methods and instruments are carefully validated. Each laboratory follows its own protocol for validation. It is recommended during the validation that 10 to 20 blanks in the same matrix be used (16). The protocols call for evaluating selectivity, linearity, accuracy (bias) and precision, lower limit of quantification, upper limit of quantification, unit of detection, stability, recovery, and robustness (16-18).

One important consideration in selecting a test methodology is clinical need and cost.

2.9   Laboratory Management

A toxicology laboratory in a modern medical center is open 24 hours a day, seven days a week. A qualified and experienced toxicologist, who generally is an MD or a PhD, manages the laboratory. It is expected to have state-of-the-art equipment for analysis and be staffed by qualified and experienced technologists and supervisors to conduct analytical procedures. The laboratory works closely with local poison centers, as well as the Medical Examiner or Coroner. The samples obtained in the emergency room or patient floors are sent to the laboratory by a pneumatic tube system. If transported manually, every effort is made to maintain chain of custody of the samples. Consultation with medical personnel as well as clinical toxicologists is maintained to obtain as much clinical information as possible about the patient. If the patient is unresponsive, a pathology resident is sent to the floor to talk to the person present with the patient. Every sample that is analyzed by a technician is reviewed by a supervisor, who ratifies the result. Finally, a toxicologist in charge of the laboratory signs every result. When in doubt, a sample may be sent to another certified laboratory to confirm and cross check the result.

Police officers always call to obtain information about a patient when he or she was involved in an accident or arrested for DUI or substance abuse. The police would like to talk to the toxicologist to convert serum alcohol to blood alcohol or blood alcohol to serum alcohol. The police, the attorneys, or sometimes the patient or relatives would like to know the dissipation rate of alcohol or drugs from the body. A toxicologist can give this information without disclosing a patient's name to maintain the patient's confidentiality. The results are expected to be given out only to the concerned doctor or the designated clinical personnel. There will always be instances where someone tries to impersonate a doctor to obtain a patient's results on alcohol or drugs of abuse. In such cases, it is prudent to ask for a phone number where you can call back later. It is found that the impersonator usually backs off and does not give a phone number.

It is useful to write down the conversations you had with anyone whether on private business or official business. There should be two separate notebooks—one for your personal and private phone conversations with family and friends, and the other for official business, such as phone conversations with doctors, clinical staff, police officers, lawyers, or district attorneys. A toxicologist should show extreme patience in the face of verbal abuse or profanities thrown at him from an angry and frustrated person who could not obtain results. One should remember that the court and the lawyers could always subpoena laboratory records, including the notebook that contained conversations, and samples released with details. Even though a particular test was done by doctor's orders for patient management, the result may turn out to have forensic consequences later. The legal department of the organization where you work is always of help to guide you and the laboratory staff. In large medical centers, a toxicologist is always available for consultation. In case of policy issues, such as sample release, the laboratory director or the administrator's on-call advice is obtained and recorded in the official notebook.

2.10 Words of Experience

A client's defense team, including toxicologists, pathologists, and other biomedical scientists, and the attorney representing the client, may look at the opposing toxicologist's report. A good toxicology report is expected to contain citations and references to back up the toxicologist's opinions. It is not enough for the toxicologist to throw his weight around saying that he is board certified. In this chapter, many details are given about laboratory operations. First, determine if a laboratory is certified and accredited. Does the lab participate in PT testing done by CAP and the state? How did the laboratory perform in previous PT challenges? QC is an important issue. Look into the performance of controls in a particular run. How did the laboratory perform in the previous inspections? Was there a consistent pattern of Phase II violations? Does the laboratory still use a method that is known to give false positive, false negative, or inconsistent results?

References

1. Armbruster, D.A., Dasgupta, A., Earley, R.J., Jortani, S.A., Marcus, W., and Rheinheimer, D.W. Toxicology and drug testing in the clinical laboratory; approved guidelines, 2nd ed. CLSI document. Clinical and Laboratory Standards Institute, Wayne, PA, 2007.
2. Flanagan, R.J. Developing analytical toxicology services: principal and guide. A report prepared for the international program on chemical safety, WHO/ILO/UNEP, 2005, 1–36.
3. CLIA 88. Federal Register, Vol. 57, 1992.
4. FDA. Medical Devices, Guidance and Regulations Clinical Laboratory Amendments, http://www.fda.gov/Medical Devices//DeviceRegulationandGuidance/default.htm.
5. Medicare, Medicaid, and CLIA Programs; Clinical Laboratory Improvement Amendments of 1988. Sec. 353. Public Health Service Act. www.cdc.gov/clia/docs/fr02my00n.htm

6. CAP Guidelines. Procedure Manual. http://www.online-/learning.com/demos/sample/sec_14.htm
7. Procedure Manuals: Clinical Laboratory Technical Procedure Manual. 3rd ed. Approved Guidelines GP2-A3, 1996. http://www.online-/learning.com/demos/sample/sec_13.htm
8. Pennsylvania Department of Health, Division of Chemistry and Toxicology. Proficiency testing. http://www.portal.state.pa.us/portalserver.pt/community/laboratories/14158/toxicology_testing/and_approved_programs/615215.
9. Jatlow, P. Proficiency testing in clinical toxicology: An overview. *J. Anal. Toxicol.* **1**:109–110, 1977.
10. Walberg, C.B. Proficiency assessment programs in toxicology. *J. Anal. Toxicol.* **1**:105–108, 1977.
11. Centers for Disease Control and Prevention. CLIA Subpart 1, Sec. 493.937—Toxicology, http://cdc.gov/clia/regs/subpart_i.aspx.
12. Moyer, T.P. and Shaw, L.M. Terapeutic drugs and their management. In: *Tietz Textbook of Clinical Chemistry and Molecular Biology*, 4th ed. Carl A. Burtis, Edward R. Ashwood, and David E. Burns, Eds. W.B. Saunders Company, Philadelphia, PA, 2006, chap. 33.
13. Ball, S. Quality control in the clinical lab. *Clinical Lab Products* http://clpmag.com/issues/articles/2009-07_02.asp.
14. Westgard, J.O. and Klee, G.G. Quality management. In: *Tietz Textbook of Clinical Chemistry and Molecular Biology*, 4th ed. Carl A. Burtis, Edward R. Ashwood, and David E. Burns, Eds. W.B. Saunders Company, Philadelphia, PA, 2006, chap. 19.
15. Linnet, K. and Boyd, J.C. Selection and analytical evaluation of methods. In: *Tietz Textbook of Clinical Chemistry and Molecular Biology*, 4th ed. Carl A. Burtis, Edward R. Ashwood, and David E. Burns, Eds. W.B. Saunders Company, Philadelphia, PA, 2006, chap. 14.
16. Dadger, D. and Bennet, P.E. Evaluation of bio-analytical selectivity and drug stability. *J. Pharm. Bio. Ed. Anal.* **14**:23–31, 1995.
17. Peters, F.T., Drummer, O.H., and Musshoff, F. Validation of new methods. *Forensic Sci. Int.* **165**:216–224, 2007.
18. Scientific Working Group on Forensic Analysis of Chemical Terrorism (SWGFACT). Validation guidances for laboratories performing forensic analysis of chemical terrorism. *Forensic Sci. Comm.***7**:1–14, 2005.

Unexpected and Unusual Results; Unusual Requests

3

In this chapter, a brief description of unusual and unexpected results is given. These do happen in busy clinical toxicology laboratories and are not unique to any one laboratory. Most of these results were published in peer-reviewed scientific journals. Unusual results include:

1. False-positive serum ethanol levels
2. Attempted suicide by chloroform
3. Acute ethanol intoxication in a 7-month-old infant
4. Carry-over cocaine
5. Nonalcoholic beer and blood alcohol levels
6. Attempted suicide by phenylbutazone
7. Other unusual requests

3.1   False-Positive Serum Ethanol Levels

In the clinical toxicology laboratory, approximately 40% of the workload is usually serum alcohols and the remaining workload deals with drug screens, volatiles, other therapeutic drugs, over-the-counter drugs, and plant and animal toxins. GC is the gold standard for serum/blood alcohol determination. However, to determine serum alcohols in a busy medical center by GC is slow, costly, and requires professional time of an experienced technologist (1). With the discovery of enzymatic methods of serum alcohol determination, the tests became rapid and inexpensive. Once the Food and Drug Administration (FDA) approved this method, several manufacturers came up with reagents and instruments to measure serum alcohol levels. The enzymatic method follows the reaction principle as given in the following.

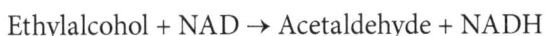

ADH
Ethylalcohol + NAD → Acetaldehyde + NADH
ADH = alcohol dehydrogenase; NAD = nicotinamide adenine dinucleotide

The machine measures absorbance of NADH generated at wavelengths of 340 nm. An increase in absorbance due to NADH is proportional to ethyl alcohol concentration in the sample. Using the enzymatic method developed

15

by Syva Company, Palo Alto, California on Cobas Mira S instrument, ethyl alcohol determinations were carried out (2).

Problems began to appear in pediatric patients from a children's hospital. The first patient was a four-month-old boy with postnatal respiratory problems. He developed cardiopulmonary arrest due to upper respiratory infections. A serum sample obtained in the emergency department gave a serum alcohol of 105 mg/dL by the enzymatic method. Headspace GC did not detect any alcohol.

The second patient was a two-month-old girl born to a mother with a history of alcohol and cocaine abuse. The infant died due to cardiopulmonary arrest. Enzymatic serum ethanol determination gave an alcohol level of 60 mg/dL. GC determination did not detect any alcohol.

When these sera samples were retested, the same results were obtained—positive by enzymatic method and no alcohol by GC. The cause for a false-positive alcohol reading by the enzymatic method and no alcohol by GC was investigated. The same sera samples were retested by other enzymatic methods with a different instrument. Identical results were obtained—positive serum ethanol by enzymatic method and no serum ethanol by GC. The possibility that another endogenous enzymatic reaction that converts NAD to NADH might generate falsely elevated alcohol readings was investigated. One such possible interfering reaction appeared to be

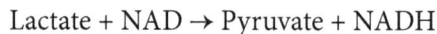

$$\text{LDH}$$
$$\text{Lactate} + \text{NAD} \rightarrow \text{Pyruvate} + \text{NADH}$$
$$\text{LDH} = \text{Lactate dehydrogenase}$$

To confirm this possibility, a series of experiments was performed by obtaining serum samples from a number of autopsy subjects. Lactate and LDH enzyme activity levels and alcohol levels were determined in these sera samples. Alcohol levels were determined by four different methods. They are Abbot, Roche, Syva, and GC. Serum samples from healthy volunteers were obtained and their LDH and lactate levels were determined. Samples were spiked with increasing concentrations of LDH and lactate and tested for alcohol levels by GC, Abbot, Roche, and Syva methodologies. These experiments proved that lactate and LDH present in the serum give falsely elevated ethanol levels but not by GC (3).

Published reports in the scientific literature show that elevation of lactate and LDH occurs in postmortem serum samples and in sera of trauma and injuries, immune-compromised patients, and patients with systemic fungal infections. In these cases, it is useful to check ethanol levels by headspace GC. In case of automobile accidents involving severe traumas, both lactate and LDH increase and the elevated lactate does not clear rapidly (1,3–5). If the victim is transported by an ambulance to the hospital, the paramedics may give IV Lactate–Ringer solution. This is another factor in the elevation of lactate on top of already elevated LDH. Under these circumstances, false-positive ethanol occurs if the laboratory measures serum alcohol levels by an enzymatic method utilizing ADH and NAD. Even if the controls and calibrators work, the enzymatic method still can give falsely elevated alcohol levels due to the presence of LDH and lactate.

3.2 Chloroform Poisoning

The next interesting case is a suicide attempt using chloroform. The effects of chloroform ($CHCl_3$), carbon tetrachloride (CCl_4), and other hydrocarbons on small experimental animals like mice and rats are well studied. In the earlier medical literature, the use of CCl_4 to treat intestinal helminthic infestations was indicated (6). CCl_4 is no longer used in human medicine because of its toxicity. A suicide attempt by chloroform provided a rare opportunity to study its effects in humans.

A 33-year-old Caucasian female who worked in a dentist's office injected herself intravenously with 0.5 ml of chloroform. She became unconscious, but woke up the next morning and realized that she was not dead. She then drank about half a cup of chloroform and became unconscious but woke up several hours later. She vomited and became unconscious again. She was found unresponsive on the kitchen floor. She was brought to the emergency room, and was found to be alert and in no apparent distress.

She was treated with hyperbaric oxygen, cimetadine, and N-acetylcysteine. Analysis of chloroform in her blood was done by headspace GC (Figure 3.1). Her sequential serum samples were analyzed daily for up to 11 days to monitor her liver necrosis, liver function, and liver regeneration. Markers for liver necrosis are alanine aminotransferase, units/dL (ALT), aspertate aminotransferase, units/dL (AST), lactate dehydrogenase, units/dL (LDH), and alkaline phosphatase, units/dL (ALP). Biomarkers for liver function are total bilirubin (TBIL), direct bilirubin (DBIL), prothrombin time (PT), and activated partial prothrombin time (APTT). The markers for liver regeneration including γ-glutamyl transferase (GGT), α-fetoprotein (AFP), des γ-carboxy prothrombin (DCP), and retinol-binding protein (RBP) were quantitated (7). The values were divided into three groups:

1. Markers for liver necrosis
2. Markers for liver function
3. Markers for liver regeneration

The values were normalized and the averages of these values were plotted for each day, up to 11 days (Figure 3.2). From the graph, it is obvious that liver

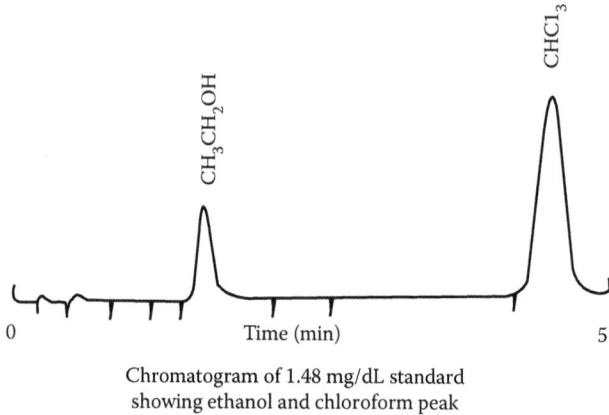

Chromatogram of 1.48 mg/dL standard
showing ethanol and chloroform peak

Figure 3.1 Chromatogram of 1.48 mg/dL standard showing ethanol and chloroform peaks. (Reprinted with permission from *Journal of Analytical Toxicology*.)

necrosis peaked by day four and declined rapidly, with a steady and consistent increase in liver regeneration. The liver regeneration remained steady throughout 11 days of observation. A social worker talked to the patient and she was then transferred to psychiatric care. When the woman's condition improved, liver necrosis decreased, and liver function was stabilized, she was then discharged (**8**).

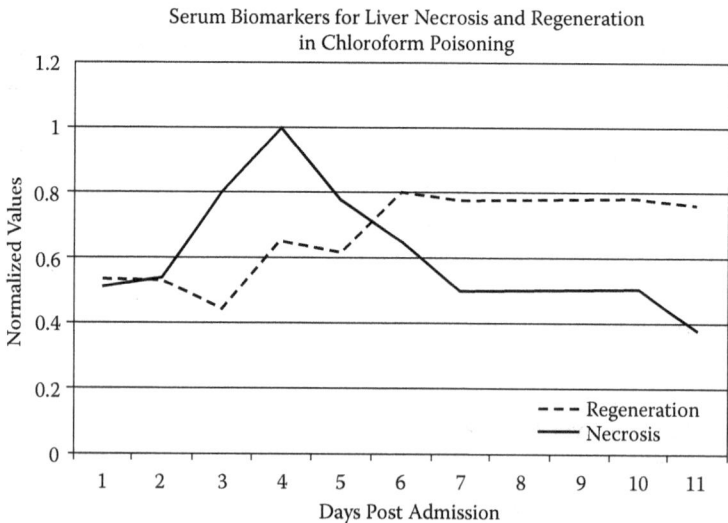

Figure 3.2 Serum biomarkers for liver necrosis and regeneration in chloroform poisoning. (Reprinted with permission from *Journal of Analytical Toxicology*.)

3.3   Acute Ethanol Intoxication in a 7-Month-Old Infant

A 7-month-old infant who accidentally ingested alcohol provided a unique opportunity to make observations on the elimination of ethanol in infants (**9**). There were no such reports in the scientific literature.

A female baby weighing 10.9 kg was brought to the emergency room by her grandmother, who accidentally mixed baby formula with unknown amount of vodka. After feeding the baby with this formula, the infant became hyperactive and behaved strangely. The baby vomited two times and the grandmother smelled alcohol in the emesis. The baby was brought to the emergency room, and the infant was noted to be active and alert. The baby was not in respiratory distress and was not irritable. The infant's vital signs were normal. A stat serum ethanol was ordered. Infusion of normal saline was started. The baby was transferred to the nursing unit.

The serum ethanol on admission was 183 mg/dL. Subsequent ethanol levels in serum at 1 hour 45 minutes and at 8 hours 5 minutes were 96 mg/dL and no detectable amount, respectively. Vodka has 40% alcohol. Considering the baby's weight and the volume of distribution for ethanol, it is calculated that the infant ingested 47.45 ml of vodka.

Alcohol toxicity in adults is well studied. At 50 to 100 mg/dL in blood, it causes central nervous system (CNS) depression, loss of coordination, loss of judgment, and loss of visual acuity. According to the published literature, death occurs at and above 400 mg/dL of ethanol in blood. In most U.S. states, the legal limit for blood alcohol is set at 80 mg/dL. Blood alcohol level above this is considered driving under the influence (DUI). In a normal healthy individual, the elimination of ethanol follows zero order kinetics. Approximately 20 mg/dL of ethanol is dissipated from an adult in 1 hour (**10**). Ethanol by itself causes insignificant toxicity when compared with its metabolites acetaldehyde and acetic acid. This metabolic conversion takes place due to the enzyme alcohol dehydrogenase (ADH) present in the cytosol, cytochrome P450 (CYP2E1) in microsomes, and catalase in peroxisomes. In turn, acetaldehyde is converted to acetic acid by aldehyde dehydrogenase in mitochondria (**11**). Since the infant did not exhibit any toxic effects due to the metabolites of alcohol conversion, it can be presumed that metabolic conversion of ethanol did not take place. In fact, CYP2E1 is only activated after birth and reaches 30 to 40% of the adult levels by one year (**12**). ADH follows similar developmental expression, with the infants aged 9 days to 2 months expressing 80% less ADH activity than adults. Adult activities are found after 5 years of age (**13**). These factors suggest that ethanol is rapidly cleared in infants (**14,15**).

3.4   Carry-Over Cocaine

The case is about Mrs. Roberta Chinchilla. She has history of asthma, which sometimes flares up severely. Her husband brought her to the emergency room as she developed breathing difficulties. In the emergency room, they immediately put her on oxygen and tried to stabilize her. Despite their best efforts, she developed cardiac arrest and died. The nursing notes indicated that the nurses were told that there was a party in her house in which she drank only Coca-Cola. The nursing notes instead abbreviated Coca-Cola and wrote that she had Coke at the party. Roberta was a non-smoker, but a few people were smoking at the party. After a couple of hours, Roberta developed respiratory distress, 911 was called, and the ambulance brought her to the emergency room. Stat serum alcohol and urine drug screens were requested. Serum was negative for ethanol. The urine was extracted and processed for drug analysis by GC-MS and an aliquot of the extract was drawn into a syringe and injected into the GC-MS instrument. Indeed, there were significant peaks, which were identified as that of cocaine and its metabolite. The technologist called the emergency room and talked to the nurses, and reported the presence of cocaine and its metabolite in the patient's urine. Since the nursing notes indicated that the patient had Coke, both the nurse and the technologist were not surprised to see the presence of cocaine and its metabolites in the patient's urine sample. Soon, the police got involved, visited the patient's house, and questioned the husband as well as other relatives.

The husband hired an attorney, and strongly objected to this insinuation. He contended that his late wife was a God-fearing, church-going family woman with children and grandchildren. His wife never smoked or drank alcohol. She never abused drugs. He requested the laboratory to check whether there could be a mistake in the analysis. The analysis was repeated by GC-MS after re-extracting the urine sample. No cocaine or metabolites were found. The technologist noticed that the previous sample in the run was from a patient who was a confirmed chronic drug abuser with a history of jail time. His urine was analyzed before Mrs. Chinchilla's urine sample. The urine extract of the previous sample from the drug addict had massive peaks of cocaine and its metabolite. Apparently, the syringe that was not washed enough and the same syringe was used to inject Mrs. Chinchilla's extract. This contaminated the GC-MS spectra of the patient sample. This gave a false positive for cocaine and its metabolite in the GC-MS. Since then, the laboratory introduced two syringes and made sure that each syringe was washed before and after use with a solvent.

3.5   Nonalcoholic Beer and Blood Alcohol Levels

This case illustrates that metabolism of alcohol by the liver is slowed down considerably in cases of end-stage liver disease. Several patients with liver failure request liver transplants. However, in chronic alcoholics with substantial liver pathology or deficiency of ADH, the metabolism of ethanol is substantially reduced resulting in the elevation of blood alcohol levels. With the availability of nonalcoholic beer, it became evident that some patients with alcoholic liver disease were substituting nonalcoholic beer as a way of coping with their previous habit of alcohol consumption. Nonalcoholic beer contains 0.05% of alcohol. Even this small amount of alcohol is not metabolized by patients with end-stage liver disease. This case illustrates how a patient achieved a blood alcohol level of 57 mg/dL after consuming nonalcoholic beer.

A 33-year-old Caucasian male was diagnosed with liver failure, and referred to the transplant unit as a possible candidate for liver transplant. He reported a 14-year history of alcohol abuse, drinking six 12-ounce beers every day. An abdominal CT scan showed a small cirrhotic liver. Liver volume was not calculated. On examination at the clinic, he was noted to have alcoholic breath. Although he was asked not to drink alcohol, his primary care physician allowed him to drink nonalcoholic beer. He drank six 12-ounce cans of nonalcoholic beer the night before his appointment. He also drank three more cans of nonalcoholic beer the morning before he came to see the doctor at the transplant unit. His blood alcohol that morning was 57 mg/dL. Because of the absence of ADH in the liver, the oxidation of ethanol is taken over by catalase (**14**). Nonalcoholic beer contains a small amount of alcohol and even this small amount accumulated in the blood in the absence of ADH in the liver (**16**).

3.6   Phenylbutazone Poisoning

This case illustrates the role of the laboratory in the management of phenylbutazone poisoning with a successful outcome for the patient. This drug is discontinued in human medicine because of its toxicity and suppression of bone marrow. However, this drug is still used as a painkiller in veterinary medicine. Upon oral administration, the drug is rapidly absorbed and is protein bound. Peak drug levels in serum occur in 2 to 8 hours. It is eliminated mostly through urine. This drug is hepatotoxic as well as nephrotoxic (**17**).

This investigation employed a strategy for the identification of the drug and used a unique approach to estimate the amount of drug in serum and its elimination over a period of time during successful detoxification of the patient. Biomarkers for liver necrosis and liver regeneration were determined in sequential serum samples to guide the therapeutic approach in the management of a patient who tried to commit suicide (7). Brief details are given in the following case.

A 15-year-old female patient was brought to the emergency room of a community hospital. She was later transferred to a children's hospital. According to her family, the patient was found unresponsive near her bed. A few of minutes later, the patient had a seizure that lasted approximately one minute. It was reported that the patient had bluish discoloration of her lips. There were no empty bottles or pills in the room or near her bed. A sample of her urine was sent to the laboratory for drug screens, as well as for comprehensive drug screen determination.

The urine was negative for drugs of abuse. The comprehensive drug screen analysis by GC-MS showed the presence of several peaks and a peak identified as phenylbutazone. The physician taking care of the patient presented these findings to the mother. The mother told the doctor that the patient was involved in a fight with her classmates the previous day and was very upset. The patient helps in the family farm and takes care of horses. They give phenylbutazone to the horses to alleviate pain. The mother could not tell whether any tablets were missing. Clinical management of the patient included treatment for respiratory and cardiac depression. In addition, the clinicians focused on detoxifying the patient. Plasmapheresis was started on Day 3 of her admission. The patient regained consciousness and her condition improved considerably. The patient fully recovered by Day 7 and was discharged to psychiatric care.

The patient had acute renal failure and there was biochemical evidence for liver necrosis. Enzyme-multiplied immunoassay technique (EMIT) was used for drug screens in urine. On the day of admission, urine was found to be negative for normally abused drugs. Serum comprehensive drug screen by GC-MS showed several major and minor peaks. One major peak was identified as phenylbutazone by spectral library. The peak areas of internal standard, barbital, and that of phenylbutazone were measured and calculated ratios of phenylbutazone to barbital showed a decline from Day 3 to Day 7 post-admission, suggesting that plasmapheresis was effective in detoxifying the patient. These results are shown in the following table.

Day (Post-Admission)	Peak Area of Control (A)	Peak Area of Drug (B)	Ratio (A/B)
3	179439009	42960031	4.2
5	49439734	22199712	2.2
6	11447700	22274784	0.5
7	17874160	24704758	0.7

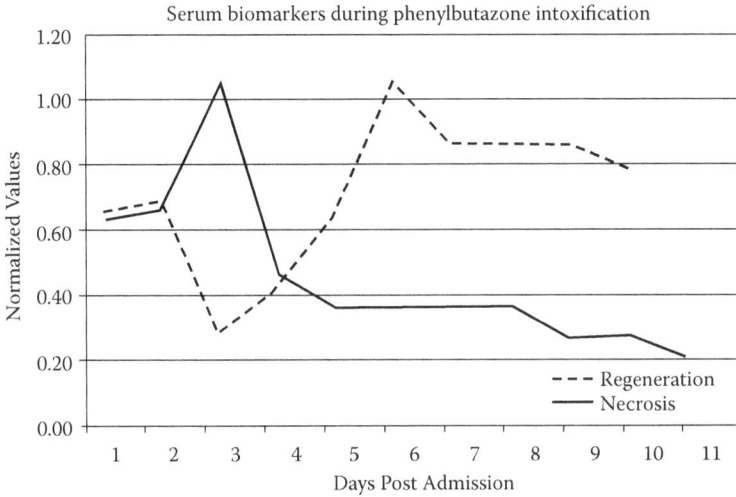

Figure 3.3 Serum biomarkers during phenylbutazone intoxificaiton. (Reprinted with permission from *Journal of Toxicology Clinical Toxicology.*)

Serum biomarkers were measured in sequential samples every day, starting on Day 3 as shown earlier in the chloroform poisoning case. ALT and AST were selected for liver necrosis, and des γ-carboxy prothrombin (DCP), α-fetoprotein (AFP), and gamma glutamyl transpeptidas (GGT) were selected for liver regeneration. The values were normalized and markers for necrosis were grouped together. Similarly, the values for markers of liver regeneration (Figure 3.3) were grouped together and plotted against the day of admission (7). From the graph, it is apparent that by Day 4, liver necrosis declined and regeneration of the liver increased steeply. These findings show that it is possible to predict the outcome of a patient from acute liver toxicity by measuring the biomarkers in the sequential serum samples (**18**).

3.7   Unusual Requests

A toxicology laboratory in a modern medical center deals with unusual requests. Here is an example.

Two young women work in a human resources department. Sandy lives in Elizabeth Township and drives to work. She is paranoid about pollution and the presence of contaminants in the city water supply. She brings her own water from a well in her backyard. She keeps this water in a tightly closed jug and keeps it under her desk. The other young woman is Barbara who lives in the city with her parents. She comes to the office by local bus, and eats her lunch in the cafeteria. Sandy and Barbara argue with each other all the time. Not only are they not friends, they actually hate each other. Sandy went to their supervisor and complained that the water she brings from her home does not smell or taste good. In fact, Sandy suspects that Barbara might be urinating in her jug of water when Sandy is away from her desk. The section supervisor called the toxicology laboratory and asked them to determine whether the water in Sandy's jug was contaminated with urine. The absence of creatinine in the drinking water in the jug ruled out urine contamination.

Sometimes the laboratory may be asked to determine whether IV bags are tampered with or whether there is any suspicious dilution of narcotic pain medications. Suspicious syringes found in patients' rooms or doctors' offices are brought in to have the contents identified.

References

1. Burtis, C.A., Ashwood, E.R., and Burns, D.E. (Eds.) *Tietz Textbook of Clinical Chemistry and Molecular Biology*, 4th ed. W.B. Saunders Company, Philadelphia, PA, 2006.
2. Jortani, S.A. and Poklis, A. EmitETS plus ethyl alcohol assay for the determination of ethyl alcohol in human serum and urine. *J. Anal. Toxicol.* **16**:368–371, 1992.
3. Nine, J.S., Moraca, M., Virji, M.A., and Rao, K.N. Serum-ethanol determination: Comparison of lactate and lactate dehydrogenase interference in three enzymatic assays. *J. Anal. Toxicol.* **19**:192–196, 1995.
4. Abramson, D., Scales, T.M., Hitchock, R., Troooskin, S.Z., Henry, S.M., and Greenspaan, J. Lactate clearance and survival following injury. *J. Trauma* **35**:584–590, 1993.
5. Didwania, A., Miller, J., Kassel, D., Jackson, E.V., and Chernow, B. Effect of lactated Ringer's solution infusion on the circulating lactate concentration: Part 3. Results of respective, randomized, double-blind, placebo-controlled trial. *Crit. Care Med.* **25**:1851–1854, 1997.
6. Lamson, P.D. and Ward, C.B. Chemotherapy of helminthic infestations. *J. Parasitol.* **18**:173–199, 1932.
7. Rao, K.N., Virji, M.A., Moraca, M.A., Diven, W.F., Martin, T.G., and Schneider, S.M. Role of serum markers for liver function and liver regeneration in the management of chloroform poisoning. *J. Anal. Toxicol.* **17**:99–102, 1993.
8. DiMaio, V.J. and DiMaio, D. *Forensic Pathology*, 2nd ed. CRC Press, Boca Raton, FL, 2001, pp. 516–519.
9. Kavet, R. and Nuss, K. The toxicity of inhaled methanol vapor. *Crit. Rev. Toxicol.* **21**:21–50, 1990.
10. Parkinson, A. Chapter 23: Toxic effects of metals. Chapter 24: Toxic effects of solvents and vapors. In: *Casarett and Doull's Toxicology: The Basic Science of Poisons*, 5th ed. Kurtis D. Klaassen (Ed.), McGraw-Hill, New York, 1996, pp. 855–906.
11. Viera, I., Sonnier, M., and Crestiel, T. Developmental expression of *CYP2E1* in the human liver. *Eur. J. Biochem.* **283**:476–483, 1996.
12. Pakkarainen, P.H. and Raiha, N.C.R. Development of alcohol dehydrogenase activity in the human liver. *Pediat. Res.* **1**(3):165–168, 1967.

13. Wu, H.B., Kelly, M.C., Ostheimer, D., Forte, E., and Hill, D. Definitive identi-fication of an exceptionally high methanol concentration in an intoxication of a surviving infant: methanol metabolism by first order elimination kinetics. *J. Forensic Sci.* **40**:315–320, 1995.
14. Chikwava, K., Lower, D.R., Frangiskakis, S.H., Sepulveda, J.L., Vrji, M.A., and Rao, K.N. Acute ethanol intoxication in a 7-month-old infant. *Pediat. Dev. Pathol.* **7**:400–402, 2004.
15. DiMartini, A.F. and Rao, K.N. Elevated blood ethanol levels caused by nonalco-holic beer. *J. Clin. Forensic Med.* **6**:106–108, 1999.
16. Flower, R.J., Moncada, S., and Vane, D.R. Analgesic-antipyretics and anti-inflammatory agents; drugs employed in the treatment of gout. In: *Goodman and Gilman's The Pharmacological Basis of Therapuetics,* 7th ed. Gilman, A.G., Goodman, L.S., Rall, T.W., and Murad, R. (Eds.), Macmillan Publishing Company, New York, 1985, pp. 674–715.
17. Baselt, R.C. and Cravey, R.H. *Disposition of Toxic Drugs and Chemicals in Man.* Chemical Toxicology Institute, Foster City, CA, 1995, p. 802.
18. Virji, M.A., Venkataraman, S.T., Lower, D.R., and Rao, K.N. Role of labora-tory in the management of phenylbutazone poisoning. *J. Toxicol. Clin. Toxicol.* **41**:1013–1024, 2003.

Serum/Blood Ethanol

4

British scientists developed a national scale to assess the harm of drugs for potential misuse. This study was published in *Lancet* (**1,2**). This study, based on physical, psychological, and social problems caused by misused drugs and alcohol, concluded that alcohol was the most harmful of the drugs that are misused. According to the scale developed by the British scientists, alcohol is three times more harmful than cocaine or tobacco. In this chapter, a brief description of the methods available for the determination of serum/blood ethanol is given. Essentially, these involve serum alcohol determinations for medical management of the patient. In the case of forensic alcohol determinations, a blood sample is required. Serum/blood ethanol levels are determined by GC, which is considered the gold standard. Several automated enzymatic methods are developed, which generally require a serum sample.

4.1 Headspace Gas Chromatograph

A variety of GCs is available in the market. All GCs operate under the same principle. Headspace GC consists of a long column packed with inert material. An aliquot of the sample of blood or serum is put in a vial that is sealed with a rubber septum or stopper and is heated. The vapors from the vial are injected automatically into the column. Vaporized compounds are moved through the column by inert gases. The compounds are separated while moving through the column. At the end of the column, a detector detects the compounds by a signal generated and gives out a peak on a chart that rolls at specified speed. The compounds are identified by the retention times. A known standard compound of known quantity mixed with a sample generates a peak. This standard peak area is compared with the area of the compound in question. The peak areas of the standard are compared with the peak area of the compound in question and are used for quantization.

A technologist using a variety of techniques such as increasing or decreasing the flow rate of inert gases, altering the temperature of the column, or altering the speed of the chart can modify the resolution of the chromatograph. GC analysis is now automated so that a technologist can load the carousel with several sealed vials with blood/serum samples and leave it in the instrument to be analyzed. With this technique, it is possible to quantify ethanol, acetaldehyde, acetone, methanol, and isopropanol. It is possible to identify volatile hydrocarbons present in serum/blood. The reader may recall that in Chapter 3 this technique was used to identify chloroform in the blood of a patient with chloroform poisoning.

GC is considered the gold standard because false-positives generally do not happen. The method is precise and reliable. However, an experienced technologist is needed to conduct the GC analysis. The machine needs periodic maintenance, and occasionally the column needs to be repacked or replaced with a new column. GC analysis is time-consuming despite some degree of automation. For emergency rooms requiring stat analysis for serum/blood ethanols, other techniques such as automatic enzymatic assays are used. In general, because of its accuracy and absence of false-positive results, GC is the technique used for forensic purposes (3).

4.2   The Vitros Chemistry Analyzer

This instrument is made by Johnson & Johnson. It is a versatile chemistry analyzer and operates on slide technology. In addition to several analytes, serum alcohols can be measured by this instrument. Essentially, a 10-µl sample of serum is pippetted by the instrument on a test slide containing nicotinamide adenine dinucleotide (NAD), alcohol dehydrogenase (ADH), and tris(hydroxymethyl)aminomethane (TRIS). On incubation for 5 min at 37°C, NADH is generated, which is read by the instrument spectro-photometrically at 340 nm. The increase in NADH is converted to milligrams of ethanol per deciliter of serum (4).

4.3   The Axsym Analyzer

This instrument is also a chemistry analyzer capable of determining several analytes including serum alcohols. This instrument is made by Abbott. Ethanols are determined by enzymatic method utilizing ADH and NAD. As in the Vitros instrument, alcohol is converted to acetaldehyde in the presence of NAD. NAD is converted to NADH. However, NADH combines with monotetrazolium dye in the presence of diaphorase. The instrument autopipets an aliquot quantity of serum into a cuvette containing the reagents. The resultant reaction changes the fluorescence of the dye and the changes in fluorescence are read by the machine and converted to milligrams of ethanol per deciliter of serum (3).

4.4   Syva Enzymatic Assay

Syva Company, now called Siemens, also makes reagents for ethanol testing in serum, utilizing conversion of ethanol to acetaldehyde by ADH in the
presence of NAD. This coenzyme is converted to NADH by an automated
machine. The increase in the absorbance due to NADH is measured at 340
nm and converted to milligrams of ethanol per deciliter of serum. This
method was discussed in detail in Chapter 3. As stated in Chapter 3, increase
in lactate and lactate dehydrogenase (LDH) is known to give false-positive
ethanol readings. Autopsy samples and serum from accident victims with
severe injuries and trauma and sera from patients with elevated lactate and
LDH are known to give false-positive ethanol levels (4). That is why forensic
laboratories measure serum/blood ethanol by GC (5).

4.5   Blood Alcohol Concentration

Blood alcohol concentration (BAC) depends on the number of drinks, the
alcoholic content of the drink, the period in which these drinks were consumed, the time of the first drink and the time of the last drink, body weight,
sex, age, and food in the stomach. In addition, BAC is influenced by health,
medications, and co-abuse of drugs (6).

It is accepted scientifically that a 150-lb man will have a BAC of 0.025%
after drinking 1 oz of 100 proof (50%) alcohol. This assumption is accurate
under almost all circumstances (7). BAC easily can be calculated as follows.

$$\text{BAC} = 150 \div \text{Body weight (lb)} \times \% \text{ ethanol content} \div 50$$
$$\times \text{ Ounces of alcohol consumed} \times 0.025$$

One drink gives a BAC of 0.02% in a 200-lb man. Thus, after consuming
four drinks his BAC would reach 0.08%, the legal limit in most U.S. states.
Approximately 0.02% of blood alcohol is dissipated from this man. ADH
is low in infants, neonates, and females. For this reason, females generally
reach the legal limit with fewer drinks than males do.

For medical management of the patient, serum ethanol concentration is
determined. For forensic purposes, blood ethanol concentration is required.
For this reason, serum ethanol levels need to be converted to blood ethanol
levels and vice versa. The average value for a serum-to-blood ratio was found
to be from 1.04 to 1.26 with a mean value of 1.14. Therefore, by dividing
serum value by 1.14, blood alcohol concentration is obtained (6). The level of
ethanol reaching the brain and its effect on the CNS is very well correlated

with the level of intoxication (**6**). For this reason, BAC is always correlated with symptoms of intoxication.

Blood Ethanol (%)	Intoxication
1. 0.01–0.05	There is only slight physiological impairment.
2. 0.05–0.07	Euphoria; increased self-confidence, impairment of reaction responses.
3. 0.07–0.10	Impairment of reaction sponsors, attention, visual acuity, and judgment. An individual may appear sober.
4. 0.10–0.20	Increased impairment of a sensory motor activity. Reaction times, attention, visual acuity, and judgment progress to increase in drowsiness, disorientation, and emotional liability.
5. 0.20–0.30	Staggering, drunk, lethargic, sleepy, or hostile and aggressive.
6. 0.30–0.40	Unconscious and stupor.
7. +0.4	Coma, and possible death.

4.6 Alcohol and Acetaminophen

One should be aware of the danger of taking Tylenol or acetaminophen for a hangover or headache following ethanol consumption. Tylenol is an over-the-counter drug used for pain, flu, headaches, and colds. It is also present in several medications. This drug causes liver failure if more than 10 g are taken in 24 hours. The liver metabolizes both alcohol and acetaminophen. One should be aware that chronic, moderate to heavy alcohol drinking enhances the toxic effects of acetaminophen. This drug is commonly used to commit suicide. Acetaminophen-alcoholic syndrome is a major cause of liver failure in the United States. Approximately 1 to 10% abuse this drug, and 31% of alcoholics use this drug regularly. Fasting also enhances the toxicity of this drug (**8**).

4.7 Could You Be Drunk without Drinking?

Endogenous isopropanol and ethanol could occur in some people. In case of diabetic keto-acidosis, the acetone in the body could be converted to isopropanol. This isopropanol induces intoxication in the individual (**9**).

Endogenous ethanol can be generated by fungal infections. The following published case from scientific literature (**10**) illustrates the ethanol intoxication by Candida infection in the GI tract. This fungus causes fermentation of glucose to ethanol in the GI tract by acting on digested food. The ethanol so generated causes intoxication.

A 24-year-old nurse, previously in good health, developed ethanol intoxication without drinking alcohol. Over a 5-month period, she developed symptoms of faintness, nausea, and sometimes vomiting 1 to 2 hours after eating meals. Occasionally, she reported that she fell asleep during her night duty. She further stated that she fell down occasionally, even during the day while shopping. Her diet consisted of 1800 calories per day with a carbohydrate content of 78%. She complained of general malaise and faintness. What surprised her friends is that she became unconscious two hours after eating an ordinary breakfast. Her colleagues and friends complained that she had a strong smell of alcohol on her breath. The level of consciousness corresponded to stupor and these symptoms lasted for three days. She contends that these episodes became more frequent. She occasionally fell into delirium or coma. She also experienced constipation, lasting a maximum of six days, alternating with diarrhea. Her degree of intoxication decreased after defecation. The ethanol concentration in her breath was measured and shown to be 1208 µ/L. Her blood alcohol concentration was 254 mg/dL. X-ray of the GI tract revealed slight dilation of the duodenum and frequent movement of duodenal contents into the stomach. Serial cultures of the stomach juice, duodenal juice, and fecal specimens showed numerous colonies of Candida, notably in the feces. Maximum live cell count of Candida in her watery stool specimen after an episode was found to be 2.3×10^3 per gram (10).

References

1. Nutt, D. Nutt damage. *Lancet.* **375**:723–724, 2010.
2. Nutt, D., King, L.A., Saulsbury, W., and Blakemore, C. *Development of a rational scale to assess the harm of drugs of potential misuse. Lancet.* **369**:1047–1053, 2007.
3. Linnet, K. and Boyd, J.C. Selection and analytical evaluation of methods. In: *Tietz Textbook of Clinical Chemistry and Molecular Biology*, 4th ed. Carl A. Burtis, Edward R. Ashwood, and David E. Burns, Eds. W.B. Saunders Company, Philadelphia, PA, 2006, chap. 14.
4. Nine, J.S., Moraca, M., Virji, M.A., and Rao, K.N. Serum-ethanol determination: Comparison of lactate and lactate dehydrogenase interference in three enzymatic assays. *J. Anal. Toxicol.* **19**:192–196, 1995.
5. Courtney, M. Utilizing results of various blood alcohol determination methodologies in predicting intoxication. http://www.forensic-lab.com/publications/hospital.html.
6. DiMaio, V.J. and DiMaio, D. *Forensic Pathology*, 2nd ed. CRC Press, Boca Raton, FL, pp. 516–519, 2001.
7. Karch, S.B. *Karch's Pathology of Drug Abuse*, 3rd ed. CRC Press, Boca Raton, FL, 2001.
8. Draganov, P., Durrence, H., Cox, C., and Reuben, A. Alcohol-acetaminophen syndrome: Even moderate social drinkers are at risk. *J. Postgraduate Med.* **107**:189–195, 2000.

9. Bailey, D.N. Detection of isopropanol in acetonomic patients not exposed to isopropanol. *J. Toxicol. Clin. Toxicol.* **28**:459–466, 1990.

10. Kaji, H., Asanuma, Y., Yahara, O., Shibue, H., Hisamura, M., Saito, N., Kawakami, Y., and Juraom, M. Intragastrointestinal alcohol fermentation syndrome: Report of two cases and review of the literature. *J. Forensic Sci. Soc.* **24**:461–471, 1984.

Ethylene Glycol

5

In this chapter, a brief description of ethylene glycol poisoning, symptoms, and its treatment are given. Ethylene glycol is readily available and is easy to obtain. It is stored in most car garages. For this reason, accidental ingestion by people as well as by pets happens quite frequently. Thousands of exposures and several deaths are reported every year by poison centers. Ethylene glycol is the ingredient that makes antifreeze tasty. It is a colorless, odorless syrup-like alcohol that tastes sweet. It can mix easily with sodas, juices, and other sugary beverages. Pets and children are prone to lap up a puddle of antifreeze left on garage floors. Every year 90,000 animals and 4000 children ingest this toxic liquid. Several states require manufacturers to add a bittering agent to antifreeze (1). Two published cases in newspapers illustrate a mother who was wrongly convicted based on a false-positive identification of ethylene glycol and a young woman's suicide attempt with ethylene glycol.

5.1 Mechanism of Toxicity

Most of the ingestions of ethylene glycol happen in children. A small percentage of these ingestions are accidental and the rest are intentional or suicide attempts. The toxic consequences are quite severe and include renal and cardiovascular failure, brain damage, and death. The toxicity is because of the metabolites generated by ethylene glycol due to the action of alcohol dehydrogenase (ADH). Ethylene glycol is metabolized to glycoaldehyde and then to glycolic acid (glycolate), which is responsible for severe metabolic acidosis. Glyoxylate is further metabolized to glyoxylic acid (glyoxylate), which also undergoes metabolic conversion via several pathways (Figure 5.1). Finally glyoxlate is formed, which combines with calcium forming calcium oxalate crystals in many tissues and urine (2,3).

5.2 Clinical Symptoms

Ethylene glycol poisoning causes central nervous system (CNS) depression within 12 h after ingestion. The patient may experience ataxia, slurred

METABOLISM OF ALCOHOLS

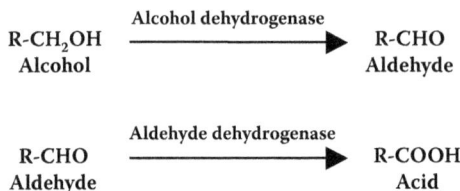

$$R\text{-}CH_2OH \xrightarrow{\text{Alcohol dehydrogenase}} R\text{-}CHO$$

Alcohol   Aldehyde

$$R\text{-}CHO \xrightarrow{\text{Aldehyde dehydrogenase}} R\text{-}COOH$$

Aldehyde   Acid

Ethylene Glycol

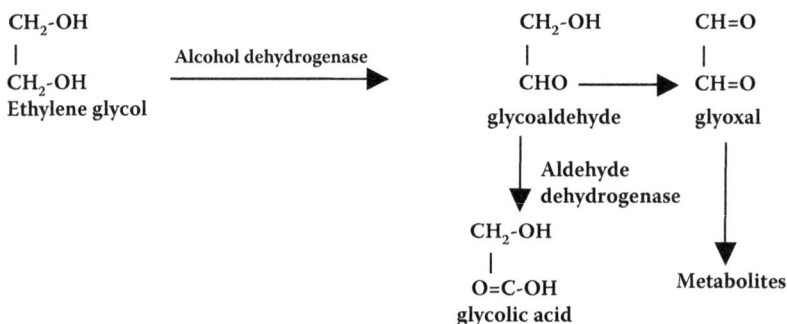

Figure 5.1 Metabolism of alcohols.

speech, and altered mental status. Anion gap acidosis and formation of oxalate crystals may also be seen. After approximately 12 to 24 h, cardiopulmonary symptoms such as hypertension, tachycardia, and heart failure may occur. After 24 to 72 h, renal failure may occur. Severe acidosis hyperkalemia, seizures, and coma indicate a poor prognosis (**2,3**).

5.3 Diagnosis

Metabolic acidosis and respiratory distress are present in most cases. Most institutions do not have the facilities to perform ethylene glycol determination. Therefore, treatment is started based on patient history and symptoms. The presence of oxalate crystals in urine and hypocalcemia are highly suggestive symptoms of ethylene glycol poisoning. Finally, the most conclusive evidence is the determination of serum and urine ethylene glycol (**2,3**).

5.4 Laboratory Monitoring

Simultaneous determination of ethylene glycol and its metabolites in serum needs to be monitored to follow the progress of detoxification. Briefly, the procedure is as follows. After serum proteins are precipitated by acetonitrile, the supernatant is derivatized by trimethylsilyl and the resulting derivatives are analyzed by capillary column GC. The internal standard is 3-bromo-1-propanol. Details of the exact procedure are published elsewhere (4).

5.5 Treatment

Where there are no facilities to monitor ethylene glycol and its metabolites, infusion of IV ethanol is started and the serum samples are sent to central referral research hospitals. Since ethanol blocks ADH, patients are treated with ethanol to maintain serum concentration of ethanol at 100 mg/dL to 150 mg/dL. This is accomplished by using 10% ethanol over a period of 20 to 60 min. If fomepizole is available, it is administered as a 50 mg/kg loading dose. This is followed by four bolus doses of 10 mg/kg every 12 h. The treatment is continued until ethylene glycol concentration is less than 20 mg/dL (2,3).

5.6 False-Positive Ethylene Glycol

This case illustrates false-positive ethylene glycol identification by two independent laboratories. It appeared that a male child died due to presumptive ethylene glycol poisoning. The mother was accused of poisoning her child by feeding the baby formula containing ethylene glycol. She was sentenced to life in prison, but while in prison gave birth to a second son who was found to have methylmalonic acidemia (MMA). On reexamination of the serum stored from the first child, it became evident that the first child also had MMA. Apparently, the two independent laboratories mistakenly identified propionic acid as ethylene glycol in the serum of the first child. The mother eventually was released from prison once the authorities realized that her first child died due to an inborn error of metabolism (5).

5.7 Positive Ethylene Glycol

This published newspaper report on the Combs trial illustrates that a positive identification of ethylene glycol poisoning resulted in Joe Combs, a Baptist preacher, and his wife receiving a sentence of 179 years in prison for child abuse. The Combses had taken a girl from an Indiana children's home, but never adopted her. This girl, Esther Combs, 19 years of age in 2007, told the police and the doctors in the hospital where she was admitted for ethylene glycol poisoning that her parents beat, tortured, and abused her. Joe Combs repeatedly raped her over the years. The doctors found both horizontal and vertical scars all over her body. The nurses, social workers, and the doctors found burn marks on her body. She had broken teeth. She could not take it anymore, so on February 18, 2007 she drank a 24-oz cup of antifreeze, brushed her teeth, and went to bed. She said she wanted to die. She was transported by ambulance to the hospital after a 911 call reported that a young woman was having seizures. This was followed by several investigations, the trial, and conviction of Joe Combs and his wife (6).

References

1. Koerner, B.I. Why is antifreeze so delicious? http://www.slate.com/toolbar.aspx?action=print&id=2103821.
2. Hall, T.L. Fomepizole in the treatment of ethylene glycol poisoning. *Cand. J. Emergency Med.* **4**:199–204, 2002.
3. Brent, J., McMartin, K., Phillips, S., Burkhart, K.K., Donovan, J.W., Wells, M., and Kulig, K. Fomepizole for the treatment of ethylene glycol poisoning. *N. Eng. J. Med.* **340**:832–838, 1999.
4. Yao, H.H. and Porter, W.H. Simultaneous determination of ethylene glycol and its major toxic metabolite, glycolic acid in serum by gas chromatography. *Clin. Chem.* **42**:292–297, 1996.
5. Segal, M. The differential diagnosis of child abuse. http://simulconsult.com/resources/abuse.html.
6. Loflin, L. Baptist preacher and wife get 179 years in prison: Combs trial. http://www.sullivan-county.com/nf0/combs/.

Drug Screens

6

In this chapter, drug screens will be briefly discussed keeping in mind different requirements between clinical toxicology concerned with patient management and forensic toxicology. The sample requirements and the methods available for drug testing are presented. The cutoff values as well as the detection periods of several drugs of abuse in urine and blood are presented. A case is presented to illustrate the usefulness of the cutoff values for drug screens. The cutoff values for drugs of abuse by rapid immunoassay techniques and for confirmations generally done by gas chromatography/mass spectrometry (GC/MS) are presented. For clinical requirements, the drug screens may or may not be confirmed, while for forensic purposes confirmations are always required.

6.1 Drug Testing

In order to identify individuals abusing drugs in healthcare, the workplace, and criminal settings, drug testing is performed. Federal government guidelines through SAMHSA (Substance Abuse, and Mental Health Services Administration), previously known as NIDA (National Institute of Drug Abuse), mandate that at least five classes of drugs be tested. These are:

1. Cannabinoids (marijuana)
2. Cocaine (cocaine, benzoylecognine)
3. Amphetamines (amphetamines, methamphetamines)
4. Opiates (heroin, opium, codeine, morphine)
5. Phencylidine (PCP)

In addition to the above-described five classes of drugs, most laboratories have facilities in place to test the following class of drugs:

1. Barbiturates
2. Hydrocodone
3. Methaqualone
4. Benzodiazepines
5. Propoxyphene

6. Ethanol
7. Ecstasy

There are five types of samples in which drug tests are performed. These are urine, blood, hair, saliva, and sweat. Among these, urine drug testing is inexpensive and quick and therefore is the preferred sample (1). Urine drug testing is also performed as a requirement for pre-employment, the military, athletics, and legal and criminal situations such as post-accident. Drug testing is useful for rehabilitation of ex-convicts, treatment compliance, and establishing the cause of death. False-positive drug tests, as well as misinterpretation of the results, have serious consequences, such as risk of prison term, loss of employment, inappropriate exclusion of athletes from sporting events, inappropriate medical treatment in emergency situations, and loss of custody of a child by the social service agencies (1).

6.2 Immunoassays

Urine drug screens are performed by immunoassay techniques and confirmed by GC-MS. Until confirmed, a positive drug result by immunoassay is designated as a presumptive positive. Generally, the hospital laboratories have several different drug screens available to the clinicians and the choice depends on their needs. Confirmations are not always necessary for the clinician for patient management. Therefore, the clinician has the choice to request drug screens with or without confirmations (1-3).

Immunoassays are cheaper and, because of automation, quite rapid. They can be used to test several samples at the same time. There are several immunoassay techniques available on the market. These include cloned enzyme donor immunoassay, enzyme multiplied immunoassay techniques (EMIT), fluorescence polarization immunoassay (FIPA), immunoturbidimetric assay, and radioimmunoassay (RIA). The main disadvantage is that immunoassays sometimes give false-positive results. For this reason, they need to be confirmed by GC-MS, which can detect small quantities of drugs. This technique is accurate, sensitive, and reliable (2, 3).

The EMIT assay principle, developed by Syva for urine drug screens, is shown in Figure 6.1.

The EMIT procedure uses the enzyme glucose-6-phosphate dehydrogenase (G6PD) tagged with a drug that retains the G6PD activity. Antibodies are made for the drug. When the enzyme G6PD tagged with the drug combines with the antibody, it forms a complex. The complex so formed loses G6PD activity. On the other hand, the drug tagged with G6PD competes with the drug present in the urine for the antibody. The antibody then forms a complex with the drug in the urine and releases the drug tagged with

Enzyme Multiplied Immunoassay
Technique (EMIT)

Drug – G6PD + Ab ⟶ Ab:Drug – G6PD   Inactive Enzyme

Drug – G6PD + Ab + Drug ⟶ Ab:Drug + Drug – G6PD   Active Enzyme

$$\text{Glucose-6-Phosphate} + \text{NAD} \xrightarrow{\text{G6PD}} \text{6-Phosphogluconate} + \text{NADH}$$

NADH generated is measured at λ 340nm and is then converted to the amount of drug present in ng/mL.

Figure 6.1 EMIT assay.

G6PD. This drug-tagged G6PD retains the enzyme activity and reacts with the substrate glucose-6-phosphate in the presence of NAD forming 6-phosphogluconate and NADH. The instrument measures NADH at a wavelength of 340 nm by a spectrophotometer, which is converted to a qualitative number indicating the presence of the drug in the urine (1-3).

EMIT drug screens can be performed with as little as 200 μL of urine. EMIT assay is quick, inexpensive, and automated (4). Many times the clinicians in the emergency room need only rapid urine screens by immunoassay without confirmatory tests. EMIT assay is known to give false-negative results (5). This technique can also give false-positive results due to interference of lactate and LDH in the urine as in postmortem urine samples (6) and in diabetes mellitus. Oftentimes urine samples are adulterated, necessitating confirmatory or alternative tests.

6.3   Gas Chromatography-Mass Spectrometry (GC-MS)

Confirmatory drug testing is done mostly by GC-MS. The method can detect a small amount of drug present in the sample. The method is accurate, sensitive, and mostly without interfering substances. However, the method is time consuming and costly, and requires expertise and the watchful eye of an experienced technologist. Essentially, the method separates several compounds present in the urine or serum by GC and the separated compounds are ionized. The ionized compounds are broken down to stable charged fragments, which can be separated further and detected by a detector. Relative abundance of a particular ion is plotted as mass spectrum as a function of mass/charge (m/z). Generally, approximately 5 ml of urine are treated with a small amount of activated charcoal and acidic and basic buffers in the presence of methylene chloride. The methylene chloride layers from the acidic and basic buffers are combined and dried. The dried extract is treated with 50 µL of methanol, of which 1 µL is injected into the instrument. In the case of serum, 3 ml are treated with 5 ml of methylene chloride. The methylene chloride layer is pulled off and dried. The dried extract is treated with 50 µL of methanol, out of which 1 µL is injected into the instrument (7). The identity of the compounds can be determined by comparing the spectra of the unknown compound with the spectra of known compounds from spectral libraries (8). Spectral libraries can be developed in-house and stored. In addition, approximately 4000 to 5000 spectra of compounds can be purchased from the Wiley Library or approximately 40,000 to 50,000 spectra of compounds can be purchased from the Pflieger Library. Spectral libraries of additional compounds are purchased when available, added to the spectral libraries, and stored in the computer. Figure 6.2 illustrates the identification of an unknown compound as physostigmine by comparing it with the spectral library.

Drugs of abuse, like any other drugs, are metabolized by the body and eventually are excreted and dissipated. The Table 6.1 illustrates the length of time drugs of abuse can be detected in blood and urine (8).

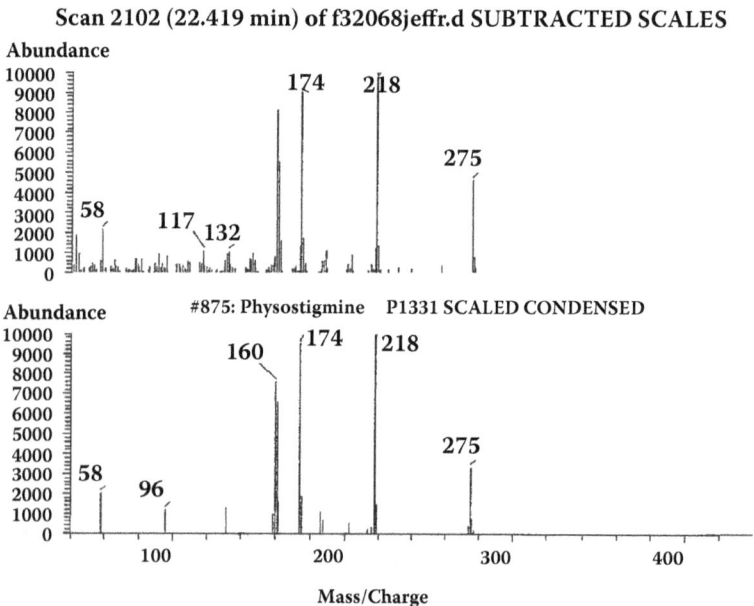

Figure 6.2 Identification of unknown compound.

Table 6.1   Detection Periods for Drugs of Abuse in Blood and Urine

Drug	Detection Period
Alcohol, ethyl	3–10 h
Amphetamine	1–2 days
Barbiturates	Up to 2–6 weeks
Benzodiazepines	3–5 days
Cocaine	5 h
Benzoylecgonine (cocaine metaboline)	2–4 days
Codeine	1–2 days
Heroine as morphine	1–2 days
Hydromorphone (Dilaudid)	1–2 days
Methaqualone (Quaalludo)	2 weeks
Methadone (Dolophene)	2–3 days
Morphine	1–2 days
PCP (Phencyclidine)	2–8 days
Propoxyphene (Darvone)	6 h
Propoxyphene metabolites	6–48 h
THC metaboline (marijuana)	
1 joint, urine	2 days
3 times weekly, urine	2 weeks
Daily, urine	3–6 weeks
Blood	8 h

Table 6.2   Immunoassay Cutoff Levels (ng/mL)

Cocaine (as Benzoylecogonine)	150
Phencyclidine (PCP)	25
Opiate	2000
Cannabinoids (THC)	50
Amphetamines	1000

Source: National Institute of Drug Abuse (NIDA), Substance Abuse and Mental Health Services Administration (SAMHSA).

In order to avoid false-positive drugs of abuse levels, SAMHSA has established workplace cutoff levels by immunoassay, as well as by GC-MS (see Table 6.2 and Table 6.3) (**8**).

Table 6.3　GC/MS Cutoff Levels (ng/mL)

Cocaine (as Benzoylecogonine)	150
Phencyclidine (PCP)	25
Opiate	2000
Cannabinoids (THC)	50
Amphetamines	500

Source: National Institute of Drug Abuse (NIDA), Substance Abuse and Mental Health Services Administration (SAMHSA).

6.4　Workplace Presumptive Positive Alcohol and Drugs—A Case Report*

Ira M. Shroud was employed as Outsource Staffer for Ordinary Personnel Services (OPS) Corporation. This is a major national company in Pennsylvania with 500 employees. This company has an employee rights manual, but it is not unionized. The manual states that an employee injured at work must submit to mandatory drug testing as soon as possible immediately after the injury. The company has a no tolerance policy for drugs, which calls for immediate dismissal if a worker tests positive for drugs.

Mr. Shroud works from 8 a.m. to 5 p.m., five days a week. He drives 25 miles each way from a nearby major city. He lives with his mother, two sisters, and their eight children. His sisters' boyfriends frequently spend the night in his apartment. Over the Memorial Day weekend, Mr. Shroud comes home to find a party in progress. The partygoers and his sisters' boyfriends are "bringing down the house." Drugs and alcohol are in use. The apartment is filled with smoke from marijuana and crack. Mr. Shroud does not do drugs but he drinks a lot of tequila.

He passes out on the sofa at 3 a.m. Tuesday morning while the party is still going on around him. He wakes up at 7 a.m. reeking from the smell of pot, crack, and alcohol. He knows that he has to drive to work, and he is short of time. He quickly changes clothes and hurriedly leaves for work.

Mr. Shroud stops at Chartwell Bagel Drive Through for his usual coffee and a poppy seed bagel, which he eats while driving to work. He realizes that he is a few minutes late. He rushes and parks his car, enters the building, and sprints up the steps to get to his desk. He trips on the last step. He hits his head on the water cooler and knocks it over, spilling water with a thundering

---

* This hypothetical case illustrates the importance of cutoff levels for drugs of abuse established by SAMHSA. This hypothetical case was used and published in the course materials for the Pennsylvania Bar Institute's Annual Workers' Compensation Program sponsored by the Workers' Compensation Section of the Pennsylvania Bar Association. Permission to use this case in this book is graciously given by Attorney Brian R. Steiner who was the program planner for the 2004 annual meeting in Hershey, Pennsylvania.

noise. His co-workers rush to the scene to help him. They call a supervisor to report the accident. Mr. Shroud has horrible pain in his head, and he thinks that both his arms are broken.

The supervisor calls for mobile assistance, and asks them to take Mr. Shroud to the company's treatment facility at the University of Marcus Hook Medical Center. He tells them to make sure that drug testing is done before Mr. Shroud gets any treatment. At the medical center's emergency room, the doctor diagnoses Mr. Shroud with severe concussion and broken arms. He also notes in the chart that Mr. Shroud smells of alcohol and marijuana.

Mr. Shroud's blood and urine are drawn at 8:30 a.m. and is sent to Sum Tymes Reliable Labs for toxicology analysis. Immunoassay performed by the laboratory indicates detectable levels of THC, cocaine metabolite, and opiates in the blood and urine. Enzymatic assay results show a BAC of 0.05%. Immunoassay for drugs in urine showed cocaine, 100 ng/mL, opiates, 250 ng/mL, and THC, 40 ng/mL.

Mr. Shroud is discharged from the hospital without being advised of his toxicology results and is asked to return to the medical center in two weeks to see an orthopedist. He is given pain medication and is asked to rest for four days and then return to work for modified duties on the fifth day. The doctor restricts him for light work with no repetitive use of the hands. On the fifth day, Mr. Shroud has blurred vision, and terrible pain in his head and arms. He calls work to tell the supervisor that he cannot drive to work. The supervisor tells him that is not necessary, as he has been fired for violation of the company's drug policy. Several days later, Mr. Shroud receives a "Notice of Denial" for his work injury from the Human Resources Department.

6.4.1   Conclusions

Based on the evidence available, Mr. Shroud's drug screens were below the cutoff levels and his BAC was also below the legal limit. Therefore, his removal from employment was not justified.

References

1. Erowid. Drug testing basics. http://erowid.org/psychoactives/testing/testing_info1.html.
2. Bowers, L.D., Ambruster, D.A., Caims, T., Cody, J.T., Fitzgerald, R., Goldberger, B.A., Lewis, D., and Shaw, L.M. Gas chromatography/mass spectrometry (GC/MS) confirmation of drugs: Approved guidelines. *NCCLS.* **22**:1–33, 2002.
3. Moeller, K.E., Lee, K.C., and Kissack, J.C. Urine drug screening: Practical guide for clinicians. *Mayo Clin. Proc.* **83**:66–76, 2008.
4. Hamilton, C.R. A rapid toxicology screen for them for emergency and routine care of patients. *Clin. Chem.* **34**:158–162, 1988.

5. Wagner, R.E., Linder, M.W., and Valdes, R. Decreased signal in Emit assays of drugs of abuse in urine after ingestion of aspirin: Potential for false-negative results. *Clin. Chem.* **40**(4): 608–612, 1994.

6. Sloop, G., Hall, M., Simmons, G.T., and Robinson, C.A. False positive postmortem, EMIT drugs of abuse assay due to lactate dehydrogenase and lactate in urine. *J. Anal. Toxicol.* **19**:554–556, 1995.

7. Ulluci, P.A., Cardoret, R., Stasiowski, P.D., and Martin, H.F. A comprehensive GC/MS drug screening procedure. *J. Anal. Toxicol.* **2**:33–38, 1978.

8. Fenton, J.J. *Toxicology: A Case-Oriented Approach.* CRC Press, Boca Raton, FL, 2002.

Plant Toxins 7

In this chapter, interesting cases due to poisoning by plant toxins are presented. The first case is about jimson weed poisoning. In addition, published articles in the popular press are also presented to highlight the toxicity of jimson weed. The second case involves castor bean toxicity. Castor bean contains ricin, one of the deadliest poisons known to humans. An interesting case published in the popular press, where ricin was successfully used to commit assassination, is presented. The third case involves mushroom poisoning, highlighting the use of serum biomarkers for liver necrosis and liver regeneration, in predicting the outcome of the patient. Excellent books are available on plant toxins and they need to be consulted for detailed study. Several drugs of abuse, such as cocaine, are extracted from coca plants. Historically, plant extracts were used by humans to kill beasts in hunting, as well as to kill enemies in war. Police can identify marijuana plants and they can identify the smell of a marijuana smoke, but they are not trained to identify other toxic plants. Emergency room physicians seek the collaboration of a plant taxonomist. Oftentimes, plants and their extracts are used to get high as they are not controlled substances, and also detection by police could be evaded.

7.1 Jimson Weed

Jimson weed (*Datura stramonium*) is a poisonous plant that originally came from the Middle East and was cultivated in England, around the 16th century. During 1676, jimson weed was grown as a potted herb to make tea and to cure asthma. This plant is also known as devil's trumpet, devil's weed, thorn apple, tolguacha, loco weed, hell's bells, devil's cucumber, and moon flower. It is an erect annual herb, farming a bush up to 3 to 5 ft tall. The leaves are soft and irregular. The fragrant flowers are trumpet-shaped, and white, creamy, or violet. The egg-shaped seed capsule is either bald or covered with spines. When mature, the capsule contains dozens of black seeds. This plant grows wild in warm and moderate regions, where it is found along roadsides, in dung heaps, and in garbage dumps. All parts of *Datura* are toxic to humans, animals, and pets. This plant may be fatal if ingested as it contains dangerous levels of toxins.

The toxic ingredients are atropene, hyoscyamine, and scopolamine, which are anticholinergic. Because of ignorance of the toxic consequences of using this plant, several hospitalizations and deaths are reported when jimson weed is used for recreational purposes. The toxic consequences due to *Datura* poisoning are complete inability to differentiate reality from fantasy. It causes hyperthermia, tachycardia, bizarre and violent behavior, and photophobia that can last several days. The antidote for overdose or poisoning is physostigmine. Even today in India, *Datura* fruit is offered in some temples of the god Shiva, and sometimes its seeds are crushed and ingested by young brides in India who are not able to withstand dowry pressures and want to commit suicide (1–4).

Treatment for jimson weed poisoning includes GI decontamination with activated charcoal and supportive care, including IV fluids, external cooling, and restraining the patient for his or her own protection. Physostigmine is used as an antidote for jimson weed poisoning (1,2,5).

7.1.1   Case Report

This case of jimson weed poisoning shows typical symptoms of anticholinergic toxicity. A 20-year-old man ingested one handful of seeds and later that day he was found on the side of the road with his motorcycle. He was agitated and confused. The police called the paramedics and he was taken to Sapota Community Hospital. At the emergency room, he was delirious and combative. He had hyperthermia with a body temperature of 102°F. The patient was given Ativan, Verapamil, and Valium. The local Sapota Community Hospital did not have physostigmine, so the patient was flight lifted by a helicopter to Anar University Medical Center.

The patient was positive for ethanol, and informed the nursing staff that he usually consumed 1/2 to 1 case of 12-ounce beers per day. He admitted that he also used marijuana and tobacco, usually about one pack a day. He had several books on subjects relating to "natural highs."

On physical examination, the patient was found to have 8-mm minimally reactive pupils. His heart rate was 123, respiration was 18, blood pressure was 160/70, and his temperature was 99.5°F. Laboratory analysis showed that L-aspertate:α-oxoglutarate aminotransferase (AST) [EC 2-6-1-1] was 103; orthophosphoricmnoester phosphorohyydrolase [EC 3-1-3.1] (ALP) was 76; L-alanine:oxoglutarateaminotransferase [EC 2-6-1-2] (ALT) was 31 and 5-glutamylpeptide-aminoacid 5-glutamyl transferase [EC 2.3.2.2] (GGTP) was 23.

GC-MS analysis of his serum showed the presence of scopolamine and atropine, confirming jimson weed poisoning. He was treated with physostigmine and other supportive measures. The patient returned to baseline health and was released.

7.2 Castor Bean

The castor bean plant (*Ricinus communis*) grows in several countries, including India. The plant contains a toxin deadly to humans and animals. The toxicity is due to ricin, which is present in all parts of the plant even though it is concentrated in the seeds. Ricin, a glycoprotein, 65,000 Da, interferes with protein synthesis (**6**). Castor oil obtained from the castor seed is a colorless to very pale yellow liquid with mild or no odor or taste (**2,7**).

Castor oil is used in the food industry. It is used as a flavoring agent in chocolate, and as a mold inhibiter. It is also used in the manufacture of soaps, lubricants, hydraulic and brake fluids, paints, dyes, coatings, inks, waxes, polishes, plastics, pharmaceuticals, and perfumes (**6**). Historically, castor oil has been used to induce labor in childbirth (**8,9**).

7.2.1 Case Report

A mother found her 20-month-old daughter playing with a package containing a mixed variety of castor bean seeds. The mother also noticed that the child had seeds in her mouth as well as several seeds scattered on the floor. The child woke up from her nap and vomited four times, producing two partially chewed seeds. As the child was behaving unusually, she was rushed to the emergency room at Palacol Research University Medical Center. At the hospital she was treated with activated charcoal and was transferred to the children's unit at the hospital 6 hours post-ingestion. The laboratory values were followed at 6 hours, 24 hours, 48 hours, and at 72 hours. These results showed that her liver enzymes were mostly elevated and came down to normal values after 3 days. The child was given supportive measurers and released.

7.2.2 Political Assassination by Ricin

Georgi Markov originally worked as a novelist and playwright. In 1969, he defected from Bulgaria, then a Stalinist state, to the West. After relocating to London, he worked as a broadcaster and a journalist for the BBC world service, the U.S.-funded Radio Free Europe, and Germany's Deutsche Welle. He criticized the Bulgarian Stalinist regime many times on the radio. It is speculated that because of this, the Bulgarian government decided to dispose of him and asked the KGB for help. He was killed on a London street after a ricin-containing pellet was fired into his leg, most likely by the Bulgarian secret police (**9**). Brief details of this assassination were published in the newspapers at that time.

When Georgi Markov was waiting at a bus stop, he felt a sharp pain in his leg and he saw a man pick up an umbrella, quickly walk away, and disappear into the crowd. He told one of his co-workers at the BBC. That evening, he developed fever, and was admitted to the hospital where he died three days later. Due to the circumstances and the statements he made to the doctors, Scotland Yard ordered a thorough autopsy. The forensic pathologist discovered a spherical ball, the size of a pinhead, in his calf. This pellet had holes in it and contained traces of ricin (**9**).

7.3   Mushroom Poisoning

Mushroom poisoning, also known as mycelium, refers to the harmful effects due to toxic substances present in a mushroom. Generally, mushroom poisoning occurs due to misidentification of mushrooms. Poisonous mushrooms contain a variety of toxins. Clinical symptoms of mushroom poisoning do not appear immediately after eating them. Sometimes, the symptoms are delayed and may appear days or weeks after ingestion. Depending upon the species of mushroom, the toxin oftentimes causes liver and kidney damage. Three of the most lethal mushrooms belong to the genus *Amanita* (**10**). There are approximately 5000 species of mushrooms present in the United States, out of which 100 are poisonous. Among these, less than 12 are deadly. Most fatalities are due to ingestion of mushrooms containing amatoxins. Amatoxin inactivates RNA polymerase II and inhibits protein synthesis leading ultimately to cell death. Amatoxin poisoning has a characteristic latent period of 6 to 12 hours post-ingestion before onset of clinical symptoms. Abdominal cramping, vomiting, and profuse watery diarrhea lead to severe fluid loss resulting in dehydration and even circulatory collapse. Once this acute GI phase is over in approximately 24 hours, the second stage begins. Even though the patient appears improved, the ongoing liver damage is occurring as evidenced by serum markers for liver necrosis and liver regeneration. In the third stage, symptoms of liver and kidney damage become apparent. With amatoxin poisoning, onset of GI symptoms typically occurs 6 to 12 hours or more after ingestion. Typically, the patient complains of severe abdominal pain, cramping, nausea and vomiting, profuse diarrhea, and weakness (**11**). Laboratory monitoring of the patient should include follow-up of biomarkers for liver function and necrosis and status of kidneys for at least 48 hours post-ingestion. The treatment, whenever possible, may include activated charcoal and maintaining fluid and electrolyte levels (**12,13**).

7.3.1   Case Report

The usefulness of serially assayed serum biomarkers for liver necrosis and liver regeneration were tested in six surviving patients of mushroom poisoning and in two non-surviving patients with acetaminophen toxicity.

Sequential serum biomarkers for liver necrosis such as ALT, AST, L-lactate dehydrogenase [EC 1.1.1.27] (LDH), and ALP alone are inadequate to assess liver damage to guide therapy or determine the prognosis in these patients when examined in isolation. A decrease in these biomarkers for necrosis could be due to a reduction in necrotic crisis or could be due to complete destruction of liver mass. Therefore, there should be a better way to guide the therapy. Six patients with mushroom poisoning who survived the liver damage and two patients who did not survive the liver necrosis due to acetaminophen toxicity are used to present clear-cut evidence that sequential analysis of biomarkers for necrosis as well as markers for regeneration indicates prognosis.

7.3.1.1   Surviving Patients

This group consists of six patients who had mushroom poisoning and were admitted to a medical center. The first patient was a Caucasian man, 44 years of age, who picked up mushrooms in the surrounding wilderness. He thought that they were edible mushrooms. He made soup out of them and ate it. The second patient was a 66-year-old white male who ate a handful of mushrooms he gathered near his house. The next four patients belonged to a Laotian family that consisted of a 32-year-old male and three females aged 41, 21, and 20. The 32-year-old male gathered mushrooms in the wilderness close to his house. The 41-year-old female made soup out of these mushrooms, which all the family members ate. The four family members were admitted to a medical center.

7.3.1.2   Non-Surviving Patients

This group consisted of two patients who went into liver failure due to acetaminophen overdose. The first patient was a 38-year-old white female with a history of depression and multiple suicide attempts. She ingested 80 to 100 tablets of acetaminophen. She was admitted to a medical center. She was treated with N-acetylcysteine, lactulose, and fluid and coagulation support. She developed acute pancreatitis and cerebral damage. Liver transplantation was not considered. Following brain death, life support systems were withdrawn. The second patient was an African American female who ingested an unknown quantity of acetaminophen tablets. She was admitted to a medical center for treatment and subsequently developed acute pancreatitis and intracranial pressure. Following brain death, her life support systems were removed.

7.3.1.3   Biomarkers for Liver Necrosis

Markers for liver necrosis are alanine aminotransferase, units/dL (ALT), aspertate aminotransferase, units/dL (AST), lactate dehydrogenase, units/dL (LDH), and alkaline phosphotase, units/dL (ALP).

7.3.1.4 Markers for Liver Regeneration

The markers for liver regeneration include γ-glutamyl transferase (GGT), α-fetoprotein (AFP), des γ-carboxy prothrombin (DCP), and retinol binding protein (RBP). Sequential serum samples were collected at several times post-admission and these biomarkers were determined. The results obtained were normalized. These normalized values are shown in Table 7.1 and Table 7.2 and plotted in Figure 7.1 and Figure 7.2.

Table 7.1   Serum Biomarkers for Liver Function in Survivors

	Necrosis Indices			Regeneration Indices		
Hours Post Admission	n	Necrosis	SEM	n	Regeneration	SEM
0–2	5	0.88	0.03	5	0.69	0.06
3–9	4	0.83	0.03	4	0.70	0.07
10–14	5	0.78	0.02	4	0.59	0.59
15–19	3	0.73	0.04	5	0.71	0.71
20–29	6	0.68	0.02	6	0.61	0.61
30–39	4	0.64	0.03	4	0.75	0.75
40–49	4	0.59	0.03	5	0.62	0.62
50–64	6	0.42	0.03	6	0.67	0.67
65–79	4	0.35	0.07	4	0.71	0.71
80–100	4	0.33	0.06	4	0.81	0.81

SEM = Standard Error of Mean; n = sample size.
©1999-2011 American Society for Clinical Pathology
©1999-2011 American Journal of Clinical Pathology

Table 7.2   Serum Markers for Liver Function in Non-Survivors

	Necrosis Indices			Regeneration Indices		
Hours Post Admission	n	Necrosis	SEM	n	Regeneration	SEM
0–2	2	0.17	0.13	2	0.94	0.02
3–14	2	0.57	0.09	2	0.7	0.04
15–19	1	0.68	0	1	0.72	0
20–29	2	0.76	0.02	2	0.71	0.06
30–39	1	0.38	0	1	0.82	0
40–49	1	0.22	0	1	0.83	0
50–64	1	0.67	0	1	1	0
65–79	1	0.14	0	2	0.68	0.02
80–100	0			2	0.53	0.07

SEM = Standard Error of Mean; n = sample size.
©1999-2011 American Society for Clinical Pathology
©1999-2011 American Journal of Clinical Pathology

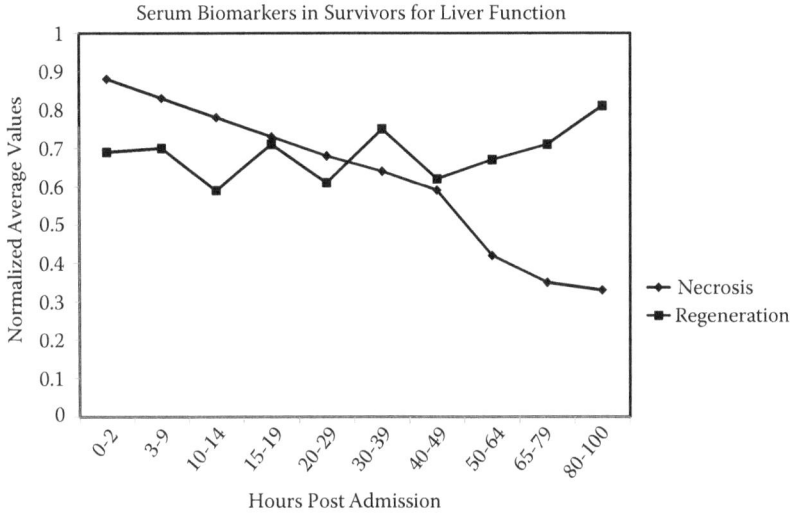

Figure 7.1 Serum biomarkers for liver function in survivors. ©1999-2011 American Society for Clinical Pathology.

From these results, it is clear that in the surviving group of patients, there is a steady decline in markers for liver macros, with a steady and sustained increase in markers for liver regeneration. This is not the case with non-surviving patients. These results clearly show the usefulness of serum biomarkers for predicting the prognosis of patients and in guiding therapy (**14**).

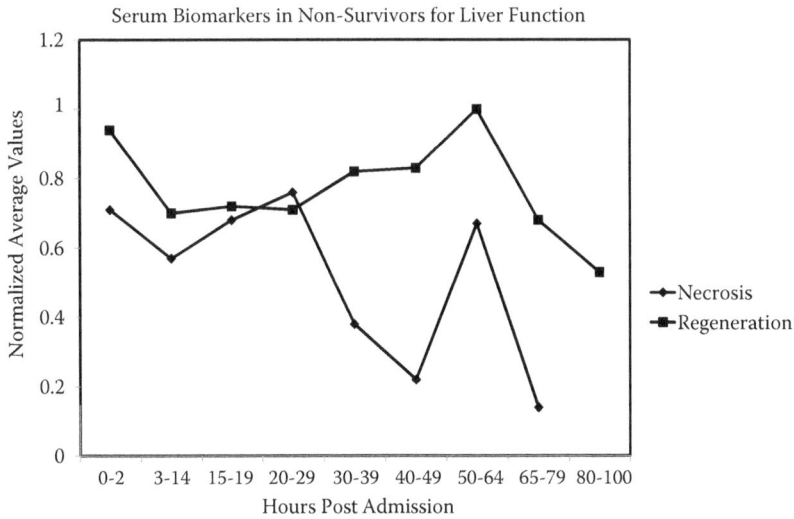

Figure 7.2 Serum biomarkers for liver function in non-survivors. ©1999-2011 American Society for Clinical Pathology.

References

1. Tintinalli, J.E. Poisonous plants. In: *Tintinalli's Emergency Medicine: A Comprehensive Study Guide.* McGraw-Hill, New York, 2005.
2. Williams, S.R., Sztajnkrycer, M.D., and Thurman, J.R. Toxicological conditions. In: *The Atlas of Emergency Medicine,* Auerbach, P.S. (Ed.). Mosby, St. Louis, MO, 2007.
3. Wikipedia. Datura stramonium http://en.wikipedia.org/wiki/datura_stramonium.
4. Wikipedia. Dowry death. http://en.wikipedia.org/wiki/dowry_death.
5. Chan, K. Jimson weed poisoning. A case report. http//xnet.kp.org/permenente-journal/fall02/fall02.html.
6. CDC. Emergency preparedness and response. Facts about ricin. http://www.bt.cdc.gov/agent/ricin/facts.asp.
7. Wikipedia. Castor oil. http://en.wikipedia.org/wiki/castor_oil.
8. Birthing Naturally. Castor oil induction. http://www.birthingnaturally.net/en/technique/castor.html.
9. Wikipedia. Georgi Markov. http://en.wikipedia.org/wiki/Georgi_Markov.
10. Wikipedia. Mushroom poisoning. http://en.wikipedia.org/wiki/Mushroom_poisoning.
11. Chang, A.K. Amatoxin toxicity in emergency medicine. http://emedicine.medscape.com/article/820108-overview.
12. Mechem, C.C. and Giorgi, D.F. Hallucinogenic mushroom toxicity. http://emedicine.Medscape.com/article/817848-overview.
13. The Merck Manual. Mushroom poisoning. www.merckmanuals.com/professional/injuries_poisoning/poisoning/mushroom_poisoning.html?qt=mushroom poisoning&alt=sh.
14. Horn, K.D., Wax, P., Shneider, S.M., Martin, T.G., Nine, J.N., Moraca, M.A., Virji, M.A., Aronica, P.A., and Rao, K.N. Biomarkers for liver regeneration allow early prediction of hepatic recovery after acute necrosis. *Am. J. Clin. Pathol.* **112**:351–357, 1999.

Animal Toxins

8

In this chapter, the toxicity of bufotenin is described. This is a controlled substance and cases are reported to the emergency room quite often. It is not possible to describe animal toxins in depth here in this book; however, excellent books and monographs are available on this subject in scientific literature. There are thousands of insects, reptiles, fish, amphibians, and other exotic animals that have venom and toxins poisonous to humans and farm animals throughout the world.

8.1 Ten Most Poisonous Animals in the World

These animals mostly use the poison or toxin for self-defense. They deliver the toxin by biting, stinging, or stabbing other animals. Poisonous animals are passive killers, while venomous animals are active killers.

1. Jelly balls jellyfish. There is virtually no chance to survive its sting unless you are treated immediately.
2. King cobra. This is the world's longest venomous snake, growing up to 5 to 6 m in length. One single bite from this animal can kill a human very easily. It is distributed in the south and Southeast Asia in dense forests.
3. Marbled cone snail. One drop of its venom can kill more than 20 humans. The venom causes intense pain, numbness, and swelling. There is no known antidote for its venom.
4. Blue-ringed octopus. This is a small animal, the size of a golf ball, but its venom is so powerful that it can easily kill a human.
5. Death stalker scorpion. Its sting is deadly to children, the elderly, and infirm, but a healthy human may survive.
6. Storm fish. Can be classified as the world's most venomous fish. If not treated within two hours, its venom can be fatal to a human.
7. Brazilian wandering spider. It is one of the deadliest spiders known and is responsible for most human fatalities from spider bites.
8. Inland Taipan, also known as a small-scaled snake. This is present in Australia and a single bite contains enough venom to kill 100 humans.
9. Dart Frog. This is present in the rain forests of Central or South America. This frog has enough venom to kill 10 humans.

10. Puffer Fish. This fish is eaten in both Japan and Korea. The skin and
some organs of this fish contain a tetrado toxin, which is deadly to
humans (1).

8.2   Bufotenin

Bufotenin, also known as bufotenine and cebilicin or 5-hydroxyl-dimeth-
yltryptamine (5-HO-DMF or 5-OH-DMF), is a tryptamine related to the
neurotransmitter serotonin. It is found in the skin of some species of toads.
Bufotenin has psychedelic effects in humans. Bufotenin was first isolated from
toad's skin during the First World War. In addition to bufotenin, the venom
of the toad also contains digoxin-like cardiac glycosides. Ingestion of venom
and eggs of the toads of the Bufo species can be fatal and some deaths have
been reported. Reports show that bufotenin containing the venom has been
used as an aphrodisiac and as a psychedelic drug. Dried skin of these toads
is smoked to get high. Sometimes such use has resulted in death. In humans,
intravenously administered bufotenin is rapidly absorbed and approximately
70% is excreted into the urine. Experiments conducted in humans show that
this has effects similar to LSD (2).

8.3   Bufotenin and Mental Disorders

It is suggested that schizophrenic subjects secrete bufotenine in the urine.
Studies have shown endogenous bufotenin is present in individuals with
psychiatric disorders and in infants with autism. Another study indicated that paranoid violent offenders or those who committed violent
acts toward family members have higher bufotenin levels in their urine
(3,4). It is reported that nialamide, an MAO (monoamine oxidase) inhibitor, increases urinary excretion of endogenously produced bufotenin in
humans (5). Serotonin and dopamine are synthesized continuously in most
animals and from these bufotenin and N-methyl tryptamine are derived
and detected in the toads belonging to the Bufo species. There are methods available for the analysis of bufotenine. Serotonin in serum can be
measured by HPLC. The normal range is 46 to 319 ng/mL. Bufotenin is
quantitated in urine by GC-MS with deuterated bufotenin as the internal
standard. The normal range is 1.8 n mol/g with a range of 0.29 to 23.2.
Psychiatric patients have 9.6 n mol/g of creatinine (6,7). The FDA placed
bufotenine on a controlled substance list (8,9).

8.4   Case Report

An interesting case was brought to the emergency room of a children's hospital. The nursing notes indicated that Mrs. Sarah Sestak divorced her husband four years ago. The couple had a handsome boy who was eight years of age. The mother had an ongoing custody battle for this boy with her ex-husband. According to the court papers, the mother gets to keep the boy during weekdays and the father gets to keep the boy during weekends. The mother lives with her mother in a small town bordering Ohio. The father lives on his farm with several farm animals and horses. There is a big lake near the farm and the boy was free to play on the farm as well as near the lake. The mother alleged that her son was playing with venomous toads found in the lake. Sarah caught hold of three colorful toads, put them in a big coffee can, and closed the can with a perforated lid. She brought the can to the emergency room. She came with her son and the grandmother. She alleged that her son was playing with the poisonous toads unsupervised. The attending pediatrician found the boy to be quite active and alert. Physical examination was unremarkable. The physician sent serum and urine samples from the boy to the laboratory for bufotenine analysis. The samples were analyzed by GC-MS and were found negative for bufotenin.

References

1. Most poisonous animals in the world. http://sciencebasedlife.wordpress.com/2011/04/12/The-most-poisonous/venomous-animals-in-the-world.
2. Wikipedia. Bufotenin. http://en.wikipedia.org/wiki/Bufotenin.
3. Räisänen, M.J., Virkkunen, M., Huttunen, M.O., Furman, B., and Kärkkäinen, J. Increased urinary excretion of bufotenin by violent offenders with paranoid symptoms and family violence. *Lancet* **324**:700–701, 1984.
4. Karkkainen, J., Raisanen, M., Huttumen, M.O., Kallio, E., Naukkarimen, H., and Virkkumen, M. Urinary excretion of bufotenin (N,N-dimethyl-5-hydroxytryptamine) is increased in suspicious violent offenders: A confirmatory study. *Psych. Res.* **58**:145–152, 1995.
5. Karkkainen, J. and Raisanen, M. Nialamide, an NAO inhibitor, increases urinary excretion of endogenously produced bufotenin in man. *Biol. Psych.* **32**:1042–1048, 1992.
6. Narasimhachari, N., and Himwich, H.E. The determination of bufotenin in urine of schizophrenic patients and normal controls. *J. Pshchiatric Res.* **9**:113–121, 1972.
7. Narasimhachari, N. and Himwich, H.E. GC-MS identification of bufotenin in urine samples from patients with schizophrenia or infantile autism. *Life Sci.* **12**:475–478, 1973.
8. What are the frogs called that you can lick and start tripping. http://www.answerbag.com/q_view/271747.

U.S. Legal System

9

In this chapter, a brief overview of the U.S. legal system is presented. The U.S. legal system consists of several layers of courts managed by the federal government as well as by state governments. Most of the scientific community, including physicians, toxicologists, and biomedical scientists, are not familiar with the way the courts function in this country. At the same time, the legal community such as attorneys, paralegals, and law enforcement personnel are unfamiliar with the workings of hospitals and laboratories. Chapters 1 through 8 deal with the medical and scientific aspects of hospitals and toxicology laboratories, as well as the way the patients are presented in the emergency room, and the way patients are treated and discharged after they get better. Some of these cases are interesting from a medical standpoint. These cases are tried and disposed of.

Generally, two types of cases come to U.S. courts for resolution. One type is criminal cases and the other type is civil litigations. In criminal cases, the toxicologists and the biomedical scientists as well as emergency room physicians are called upon to appear before the courts. The civil cases do not require the presence of a pathologist or toxicologists to appear in a court and testify, unless he or she volunteers as an expert witness. A toxicologist or a pathologist in charge of the toxicology laboratory may be subpoenaed to attend court and testify when the case comes to trial. For those unfamiliar with the operating procedures of the U.S. courts, a brief overview is presented.

9.1 A Brief Overview

Each business day, courts throughout the United States render decisions that affect thousands of people and may sometimes affect only the parties to a particular case. The law of the United States consists of many levels and is based on the U.S. Constitution. This document is the foundation for federal law, which consists of treaties and acts ratified by Congress. Thus, the Constitution and federal laws are supreme. Actually, many of the laws that guide common citizens are primarily state laws and they vary widely among the 50 states of the United States. However, most state laws cannot contradict or be in conflict with the U.S. Constitution. If Congress passes a statute that conflicts with the U.S. Constitution, the Supreme Court may declare the law unconstitutional and invalid. If any local or state court tries to enforce an unconstitutional law, the Supreme Court may reverse it. Congress enacts statutes and these statutes give power to the agencies of the executive branch to enforce them. The statutes are published in the Federal Register from time to time. Federal laws deal with the military, foreign affairs, intellectual property, aviation, telecommunication, railroads, pharmaceuticals, antitrust, and trademarks. The 50 states have their own constitutions, governments, and courts, including the state Supreme Court. Most cases are litigated in state courts. State courts deal with 27.5 million civil and criminal cases, whereas the federal courts deal with 28,000 civil and criminal cases. All states have legislative branches, which enact state statutes. In addition to the two layers of state laws, there are also local laws. States have delegated some law-making powers to townships, counties, and cities.

9.2   Civil Law

There are several stages in a civil lawsuit, mainly initiation, trial, and then possibly appeal. American civil procedure has pretrial discovery, heavy reliance on live testimony obtained at deposition or at the trial in front of a jury, and aggressive pretrial practices that might result in pretrial disposition or settlement. A civil lawsuit is initiated when the plaintiff files a complaint against a defendant alleging that the defendant has wronged the plaintiff in some way recognized by the law. In a civil lawsuit, the plaintiff requests the court to award damages to the plaintiff as a remedy for the wrongs committed by the defendant. The defendant responds to the allegations by filing an answer to the complaint in which the defendant either admits or denies the plaintiff's allegations. If the parties do not settle, then the case goes to trial. In most civil trials, the Constitution gives the parties a right for a jury trial. The losing party can appeal, in which case it may go to an appropriate court to decide on the case. The parties can sometimes take their disputes to arbitration rather than to a judge or a jury.

9.3   Criminal Law

Criminal law involves prosecution by the state for wrongful acts that are considered serious enough they cannot be deterred or remedied by lawsuits between private parties. Many of the crimes committed in the United States are prosecuted and punished at the state level. In general, the federal criminal law focuses on crimes committed against the federal government such as evading paying federal income tax, mail theft, and physical attacks on federal officials as well as interstate crimes such as drug trafficking and wire fraud. Several states consider two levels of criminal laws, one involving serious crimes and the other involving misdemeanors. Generally, most felony convictions involve lengthy prison sentences, fines, or both. Sometimes sentences also involve restitution of monetary compensation to the victim. Misdemeanors are punished by 1 year in jail and a substantial fine. Punishment for drunk driving varies widely between states as well as punishment dealing with drug crimes.

9.4   Types of Courts

There are several types of courts. The federal and state court system has two levels. These are trial courts and appellate courts. Cases are tried in trial courts and appellate courts review the decisions rendered by the trial courts. The federal courts decide on cases involving violation of federal statutes. In addition, they decide on cases if one party filing the lawsuit resides in one state and the party being sued resides in another state. A criminal case is brought by the federal government or the state government against a person for violating criminal laws. If the defendant in a criminal case is found guilty, the jury sentences him or her to a jail term, fine, or both.

9.5   Lawyers and the Legal Profession

In earlier days, there were no law schools in the United States to train lawyers. After the American Revolution, the number of lawyers has increased steadily. In 1850, there were only 15 law schools. By the year 1900, they increased to 102. Law schools then did not require previous college education. In the 1800s, law schools had a 2-year program. Currently, law schools have a 3-year program after completing a 4-year college degree. The number of lawyers has increased dramatically, and it is estimated that there are more than 95,000 attorneys in this country. Approximately 72.9% are in private practice, some in small one-person offices and some in large law firms. Approximately 8.2% work in government agencies and 9.5% work in private industries and associations. Hospitals and major medical centers have legal departments where qualified attorneys help and advise the faculty and clinicians whenever required. When hospitals do not have their own legal department, they hire law firms to help them. In case clinicians or toxicologists are subpoenaed to appear at a trial, the legal department advises them and helps them to prepare adequately for trial.

9.6   Federal and State Prosecutors

Each federal district has one U.S. attorney and one or more assistant attorneys. They are responsible for prosecuting defendants in criminal cases in federal district courts. They also defend the United States when it is sued in federal trial courts. The president appoints U.S. attorneys and they usually serve a 4-year term. The president also appoints the U.S. Attorney General and the Senate confirms him or her.

The U.S. attorneys have considerable discretionary powers in prosecuting defendants in criminal cases. They also decide which civil cases to pursue and which cases to settle out of court. In the state, persons who prosecute criminals violating state statutes are called District Attorneys. In most states, they are elected county officials. However, in a few states they are appointed. The office of the district attorney has adequate staff members and several assistant district attorneys who do most of the valuable trial work. These recent graduates of law school gain valuable trial experience by working as assistant district attorneys. Many of them later enter private practice in criminal law and others seek to become district attorneys or judges. District attorneys have a separate budget and staff members to help them. If a defendant is charged with violation of federal or state statutes and has no money, the defendant is provided with a government-appointed lawyer. These lawyers are called public defenders. In the United States, everyone has a constitutional right to be represented by an attorney. In civil cases, the issues are sometimes quite complex and for this reason, both the plaintiff and the defendant are represented by their own attorneys.

9.7   The Courtroom

The attorneys, prosecutors, and judges become part of the courtroom work group to dispose of cases efficiently and expeditiously. In addition, there are court reporters, judicial assistants, and clerks to assist in processing cases in an orderly and methodical fashion. Prosecutors strive for quick conviction of the criminal, while defense attorneys work for a quick acquittal. The courtroom work group maintains cohesion and tries to avoid uncertainty. Jury trials, in general, have uncertainty for the defense as well as for the prosecution. Finally, the courtroom work group tries to maintain the dignity of the court. The prosecutors and the defense attorney always address the defendant in a formal way. In civil cases, the plaintiff's attorney and the defense attorney address the litigants in a formal way. The litigants are to answer the questions during cross-examination briefly without unnecessary statements.

The litigants are to address the judge as "Your Honor," "Sir," or "Ma'am." The litigants always address the attorneys as "Sir" or "Ma'am." It is expected that to maintain the dignity of the court, prosecutors, defense attorneys, and expert witnesses will dress neatly and formally. The judge is called to rule upon many motions of the prosecution and the defense attorneys. The judge is also asked to rule upon admissibility of the evidence presented as well as the admissibility and qualifications of the expert witnesses.

9.8   The Jury

Common citizens are selected for jury duty and both the prosecution and the defense talk to the jurors to make sure that they are suitable to serve in that particular case. The jurors' role is mostly passive and they are expected to listen to the attorneys as well as the expert witnesses and reach a decision based solely on the evidence presented. The judge instructs the jurors about the meaning of the law and how the law applies to the case at hand. The jurors discuss the case and reach a unanimous decision. If the jury is deadlocked and cannot reach a verdict, the judge may insist that the jurors continue their deliberations until they reach a verdict. If the jury is hopelessly deadlocked, the judge may dismiss the jury and ask for a new trial. Even in a civil case, the Constitution guarantees a jury trial. Both the plaintiffs and the defendants may ask the judge to decide without a jury. The litigants may go for arbitration.

Bibliography

1. Outline of the U.S. legal system. Bureau of international information programs, 2004. http://usinfo.state.gov.
2. Feinman, J.M. *Everything You Need to Know About the American Legal System.* Oxford University Press, New York, 2006.
3. Bonfield, L. *American Law and the American Legal System in a Nutshell.* Thompson/West, St. Paul, MN, 2006.
4. Wikipedia. Law of the United States. http://en.wikipedia.org/wiki/Law_of_the_United_States.
5. Radcliffe, M.F. and Brinson, D. The U.S. Legal System. http://library.findlaw.com/1999/Jan/1/241487.html.
6. The American Legal System. http://quickmba.com/law/sys/.

Toxicology Report 10

In this chapter, the importance of writing a toxicology report and the process a toxicologist has to go through to write such a report is presented. The toxicology report becomes important when the laboratory analysis done on a patient's samples is requested by the prosecution later. The patient may be charged in a criminal case and the case comes to trial with a time lapse of several years. When a toxicologist volunteers as an expert witness and is retained by an attorney in a criminal or civil case, the toxicology report is quite a useful tool to prepare for deposition or a trial. Moreover, an attorney may present the report as evidence at the trial. The opposing lawyer may ask for a report from the expert toxicologist if one is retained.

10.1 The Process of Laboratory Analysis

A clinical toxicology laboratory routinely analyzes body fluids or other samples on several hundreds of patients at the request of physicians in the emergency room. In addition, several hundreds of samples sent from physicians from other departments as well as from surrounding hospitals are analyzed. These results are reported back to the physicians by the technologist after review by the supervisor. The results are then put in the computer and become accessible to the concerned clinical staff and physicians. The toxicologist again verifies and signs them out. If necessary, the residents rotating in the toxicology laboratory visit the patients' floors, talk to the patient or the family, and submit a report back to the laboratory, which is stored and becomes available to be retrieved. In a busy hospital or medical center, the hard copies of patients' results are stored for up to 10 years to be retrieved if and when necessary. Each hospital has its own way of storing these hard copies and in some medical centers, the records are sent to organizations like Business Medical Records for storage. Patients' samples are stored in walk-in refrigerators or freezers for up to three months. Frozen tissue samples as well as paraffin blocks are also stored. The stored patients' samples are shared or given to a coroner or medical examiner. If the samples are split, then the split samples are stored for up to 10 years as these cases may go to trial. Similarly, samples received from outside institutions for analysis are also stored. Sometimes the patients' samples are also sent to another laboratory to confirm and verify the results.

10.2　Criminal Prosecution

When a former patient is going to be prosecuted, usually the District Attorney's Office makes a phone call or sends summons by a police officer, through the U.S. Postal Service, or through a courier. By whatever means the summons is served, it is clearly addressed to the toxicologist who signed out the results. The summons needs immediate attention. A summons states the patient's name, the criminal violation of the state statutes, and the trail date, time, the courtroom, and the name of the judge expected to preside over the case. It could also state which laboratory records to bring to the trial. It is always prudent to consult Risk Management in the hospital who will talk to the District Attorney's Office to postpone the trial in case it conflicts with a previous commitment for the toxicologist. Risk Management also negotiates with the District Attorney's Office if the demands pose an unusual hardship for compliance. Sometimes the attorney representing a defendant may get a court order demanding copies of laboratory records pertaining to the patient. Even in this case, Risk Management will be of great help to negotiate with the defendant's attorney to avoid unusual demands.

Once the patient's name, date of patient's admission, and date of analysis of the patient's samples are known, a toxicologist should retrieve the patient's records from the computer.

The physician and nursing notes need to be reviewed and studied carefully. This process forms the basis for writing a toxicology report and for understanding the case a toxicologist needs to prepare for the trial.

10.3　Consultant Toxicologist and Expert Witness

There is always a demand for an experienced toxicologist. The name, place of work, and telephone numbers of a toxicologist become public record. Attorneys dealing with civil or criminal cases can contact a toxicologist to work with as a consultant. This consultation becomes a private matter outside the official duties of a toxicologist managing a clinical toxicology laboratory. Generally, university medical centers allow 20% of a toxicologist's time for private consulting work. In such an event, it is necessary to obtain written permission from the chair of the department or the medical director of the laboratories. There are also professional organizations that keep a list of toxicologists and supply the contact information to attorneys looking for experienced toxicologists as expert witnesses. This service is free for the attorneys, but a toxicologist signs a contract to give a certain percentage of fees received from attorneys to these professional organizations. A toxicologist sometimes gets a retainer and negotiates fees for reviewing the records, writing a toxicology report, and giving testimony at a deposition and trial. Travel expenses including hotel stays are also negotiated in advance. A written agreement for fees for services is obtained from the attorney. An attorney usually approaches a toxicologist requesting him or her to appear at a trial with adequate time for preparation. The toxicologist should make sure that there is no conflict of interest or violation of professional ethics. The toxicologist should not work against the institution where he or she is employed including associated sister institutions. A toxicologist obtains key documents to understand the scientific issues and leads in the case. If a toxicologist does not have the training and experience in the subject matter pertaining to the case in question, then he or she should not agree to work on that case. A toxicologist should not be tempted if enticed with money to appear for a trial at short notice. He or she should have the attorney supply all the documents about the case including the opposing toxicologist's testimony or report.

10.4   Steps to Writing a Good Toxicology Report

Counsel requests a written report because federal courts may require them in all civil cases. A written report from an expert may help a settlement to be reached. Experts' reports are marked and introduced as evidence in court. A toxicologist must be honest and ethical, and come to conclusions based on facts and solid science, not because the attorney wants it. One must remember that the opposing side may have a report from a professional toxicologist. The report must be consistent and have conclusions similar to those written in previous reports. The opposing attorney can get copies of everything that was written before including publications as well as transcripts of previous testimonies. If there is an opposing expert's report, address all of the issues raised in that report. Proper references should be cited in the report to back up conclusions. Attorneys know the value of your toxicology report in a civil suit as they can get a more favorable settlement based on your report. The report also may help an attorney to support his or her motion for a summary judgment. The legal and scientific issues in a particular case may have different importance. One has to discuss with the attorney what issues should be addressed in the report. The length of any report varies by case. If there is a draft report, label it as such and send it to the attorney. If there are questions to be clarified from the client, ask the attorney to get the answers but never talk to the client directly. An attorney should not write the report for you or modify the opinions or conclusions in your report. An attorney may review the report for its completeness. A toxicologist has to maintain his or her credibility and represent the profession. For this reason, one should be objective. Remember that expert's reports are discoverable. Always use a 12-point font and avoid substantive mistakes, bad grammar, and spelling and typographical errors. An expert must always do research based on which the opinions are expressed with appropriate citations. Define technical terms and the abbreviations used in the report. Do not comment on the credibility of the opposing expert.

The report may contain an introduction, documents reviewed, factual background, a brief description of your qualifications, clearly stated opinions and conclusions, and references. If a toxicologist cannot change the conclusions based on the available scientific literature, then he or she should state so to the attorney in which case he may opt for a settlement. The conclusions may be stated in the beginning of the report as well as at the end. Explain the concepts and try to educate your audience. Avoid mistakes and typos in the report. Answer the challenges brought by the opposing expert with respect and courtesy. The attorney may share the report well in advance of the trial with the district attorney or the attorney of the opposing side and may submit it at the trial as an exhibit with the permission of the judge. An expert is not a client; therefore, attorney–client confidentiality does not exist. Communication between the expert and retaining counsel should be protected. Draft report and e-mail communications between the expert and the retaining attorney are discoverable by the opposing attorney.

Bibliography

1. Hodgson, B.T., Walter, L., and Perrigo, B.J. Toxicology report: a review; 1999 to 2001. 13th Interpol Forensic Science Symposium, Lyon, France, October 16-19, 2001.
2. Babitsky, S. and Mangraviti Jr., J. *Writing and Defending Your Expert Report: The Step-By-Step Guide with Models.* Seek Inc., Falmouth, MA, 2002.
3. Babitsky, S. and Mangraviti Jr., J. *How to Become a Dangerous Expert Witness: Advanced Techniques and Strategies.* Seek Inc., Falmouth, MA, 2005.
4. Weisen, J.P. Tips on writing an expert witness report. www.ipacweb.org/conf//07/.

Deposition Testimony 11

In Chapter 10, techniques for writing a good toxicology report were described. In this chapter, useful techniques for giving a good, honest, effective, and truthful deposition testimony are given. The retaining attorney may give the toxicology report to the opposing attorney. The opposing attorney may request your deposition to understand the issues involved in the case and to go over your testimony at the trial.

11.1 What Is a Deposition?

A Deposition is an oral testimony of a witness taken in an out-of-court setting. This testimony could be used for discovery purposes and could be used later during the trial in a court. In a majority of U.S. states, depositions are referred as examination before trial (EBT). The testimony is taken from the expert witness under oath and the oath is administered by an official court reporter. This official court reporter records proceedings of the deposition. There is really no difference between the testimony in the courtroom and the testimony taken at a deposition except that there is no judge presiding in the latter situation. Usually, the witness, the attorneys, and the court reporter are present. Depositions are usually conducted in an opposing attorney's office or a court reporter's office and rarely at the workplace of a witness. The trial judge will make rulings over inadmissible matters. The attorney representing the opposing side calls for a deposition to find out the facts and issues involved in a case. During deposition, only the attorney questions the witness. The person who is deposed is called the deponent. Since you are testifying under oath as an expert witness in toxicology, there will be penalties for perjury for knowingly testifying something that is not true. Whatever a court reporter records, a transcript will be made and a copy will be provided to the expert toxicologist giving a deposition testimony to make corrections if needed. Except for minor corrections, making substantial changes to answers to a specific question will seriously affect ones credibility. Because of the deposition testimony, the opposing attorney knows what you are going to say at the trial. The purpose of taking a deposition is to gather information and to find out what is going on in the case. Opposing counsel would like to know the facts, the events, and how they occurred; the weaknesses in their case; and the strengths and weaknesses in the retaining counsel's case. It is also used to confirm what the opposing counsel knows and the best legal and factual theories he or she has about the case. Depositions are very useful and may become the groundwork for preparing to go to trial. Depositions allow opposing counsel to get spontaneous and unrehearsed answers from the expert witness.

11.2 Preparation for a Deposition

A toxicologist always reviews the documents that were used and cited in the report to reach conclusions and opinions in the case. A careful and thorough review of the documents is necessary to give a good, honest, and truthful deposition testimony. Discuss with the attorney the issues that may come up during your deposition. Listen to the question asked by the opposing attorney carefully before answering. If you do not understand the question, ask the attorney to repeat it. If you do not know the answer, say you do not know. You can always refuse to answer a hypothetical question or say you do not know the answer. Answer the question without giving an elaborate explanation or justification of your answer. Remember to speak clearly and politely without getting angry. Never lose your composure. You have every right to confer with your attorney during the deposition. If you are tired, request a break. The opposing attorney has a right to look at the documents you have brought to the deposition. Finally, always tell the truth. Do not let the opposing attorney put words into your mouth. Do not be afraid or intimidated; while at the same time, do not make jokes with the opposing attorney. Be aware of a leading question and if the opposing attorney asks a leading question, take a moment to understand the question and then answer.

11.3 Civil Litigation

Depositions are mostly taken in civil cases. If the witness is not a party to the lawsuit, a subpoena must be served to give deposition testimony if he or she is reluctant to do so. The attorney who ordered the deposition usually starts asking questions at the deposition. Depositions are usually taken for no more than 7 hours in a given day. A deposition gives all litigants a window to the evidence that exists in the case. After a number of witnesses have been deposed, the litigants have enough information to predict the outcome of the case if it goes to a trial. The parties can compromise and reach a settlement, avoiding additional cost of litigation. Deposition transcripts are submitted for summary judgment.

11.4   Criminal Litigation

In the United States, depositions may be taken in criminal cases; however, each state has its own laws that govern the deposition process. If a toxicologist is working for a hospital and the case involves laboratory analysis, he or she is rarely called for depositions. However, if the toxicologist is working as an expert witness with an attorney, he or she may be asked to give deposition testimony. The depositions in criminal cases are taken from an expert witness before a trial so that their testimony can be used if he or she is not available to come to court for a trial.

Bibliography

1. Feinman, J.M. *Everything You Need to Know About the American Legal System.* Oxford University Press, New York, 2006.
2. Bonfield, L. *American Law and the American Legal System in a Nutshell.* Thompson/West, St. Paul, MN, 2006.
3. Bergman, P. and Moore, A.J. *Nolo's Deposition Handbook*, 3rd ed. Nolo, Berkley, CA, 2010.
4. Malone, D.M. and Hoffman, P.T. *The Effective Deposition Strategies,* 2nd ed. National Institute for Trial Advocacy, Notre Dame, IN, 2001.
5. Wikipedia. Deposition (law). http://en.wikipedia.org/wiki/Deposition_(law).
6. Lawyers.com. Criminal depositions: preserving witness testimony. http://criminal.lawyers.com/Criminal-Law-Basics/Criminal-Depositions-Preserving-witness.testimony.html.
7. WORLDLawDirect. How to prepare for a lawsuit. http://www.worldlawdirect.com/article/556/how-prepare-lawsuit.html.
8. McCarter, G.W.C. The purpose of your deposition is to help the other side. http://www.mccarterhiggins.com/deposition_advice.html.
9. Roth, L.M. Guidelines for giving your deposition. http://library.findlaw.com/2000/Aug/1/129259.html.
10. Giving deposition testimony. http://www.kenkoury.com/depo.htm.

Court Testimony

12

In the previous chapter, techniques for giving an effective and truthful deposition testimony were given. In this chapter, a brief description of techniques to give effective, honest, and truthful court testimony is given. Testifying in court on the witness stand is an art that can be mastered by practice and experience. It is your duty as an expert witness to give an honest and truthful opinion to the court. Doctors, toxicologists, and biomedical scientists not familiar with court procedures fear testifying in court. They fear cross-examination by aggressive lawyers. One need not be afraid if one understands and prepares adequately for court testimony. Indeed, it can be a rewarding experience. Here are some tips to help you testify effectively in court.

12.1 Expert Witness

An expert witness is a professional by virtue of his or her education, training, and experience, and has specialized knowledge in a particular subject beyond that of the average person. The court could rely upon an expert's opinion about the facts and evidence in the case. An expert witness has a legal responsibility to tell the truth to the court. Perjury by an expert witness is a punishable crime in many countries. In the United States, both sides in civil lawsuits use expert witnesses and they may give completely divergent and opposing opinions. Some experts are called *hired guns* and may express their opinions, based on junk science. Expert witnesses charge fees, which are paid by the party commissioning them. A toxicology report written by an expert witness and his or her opinions are important components of civil as well as criminal trials. Expert witnesses are supposed to prepare current curriculum vitae based on which the attorney that hired them requests the court to admit them as expert witnesses in toxicology. A toxicologist may be asked on the witness stand to tell the court all the fees and expenses that he or she is charging for writing a toxicology report and giving testimony at deposition and at the trial.

12.2   Important Tips for Effective Testimony

It is important to look, sound, and act like an expert. You should convince the jury that you are a professional and effective expert witness, a knowledgeable, experienced toxicologist, and a scientist. Before coming to the trial, study the documents and refresh your memory. Remember that the United States is composed of many different ethnic and cultural backgrounds. People may speak English with different accents. Speak slowly but make sure that the jury, the judge, and the attorneys understand you. Sometimes you may need to spell out the technical terms for the court reporter. Speak in your own words. As an expert witness, you are establishing your credibility from the moment you stand up and proceed to the witness box. State your name slowly and clearly. If necessary, spell out your name. You might have to state your past and present employment and the duties you perform. You might have to state your professional experience that designates you as an expert witness. Look directly at the counsel when you are asked a question. When you answer the question, you may speak to the jury. If you are using technical terms, try to explain in nonprofessional terms what the technical jargon means. Remember you are sworn to tell the truth and express your opinion based on scientific facts published in the scientific literature. Never exaggerate, listen carefully to the questions asked by the attorneys, and make sure you understand the questions before answering. Think before you speak and explain your answer. Correct your mistakes immediately. Do not volunteer information. Answer only the question that was asked. Dress properly to maintain the dignity of the court and to reflect your professionalism. Stop speaking if counsel has raised objections to a question or if the judge interrupts you. Do not discuss the case with anyone except with the attorney who hired you as an expert witness. Do not discuss your testimony with anyone. It is important to find out whom the other side is going to use as an expert witness. If possible, get the opposing counsel's toxicology report from your attorney. It is important to review this report before trial and anticipate questions from the lawyer representing the other side. Sometimes you are sequestered and have to wait outside the courtroom until you are called inside. Find out the time, date, and courtroom you have to go to and the judge who is going to be at the trial. Be respectful and courteous. Address the judge as "Your Honor." Address the lawyers as "Sir" or "Ma'am." Try to keep the interest of the jurors in what you are saying and keep them focused on every word you say. Your body language and gestures can be persuasive. Your posture, how you sit in the witness chair, and how you speak are all important. This is particularly important during cross-examination by an aggressive attorney. After your testimony is over, wait until you are excused from the witness stand. Make sure that your testimony is over and you will not be called in again before you leave the courtroom. Generally, the attorney who hired you pays your fees before the trial or he or she may mail you a check later.

12.3   Cross-Examination

Cross-examination can be very tricky and can make you appear feeble-minded if you are unprepared. The opposing lawyer's questions sometimes are designed to catch you off guard and discredit your testimony. Ambiguous questions are designed with double meaning so that no matter how you try to answer, it can be turned around and used against you. If this happens, ask the attorney to rephrase the question before you try to answer. The lawyer can also ask a two-part question where one part is true and the other part is false. This type of question is difficult to answer and you will be caught in a difficult situation. If this happens, answer only the first part and wait so that the lawyer has to redirect the second part of the question to you. Do not take things personally and remember that an aggressive lawyer who is cross-examining has nothing against you. Personal opinions and conclusions are irrelevant and have no place in the courtroom. Simply state that your opinions are based on your education, experience, and knowledge of the published medical and scientific literature.

Bibliography

1. Feinman, J.M. *Everything You Need to Know About the American Legal System.* Oxford University Press, New York, 2006.
2. Bonfield, L. *American Law and the American Legal System in a Nutshell.* Thompson/West, St. Paul, MN, 2006.
3. Outline of the U.S. legal system. Bureau of international information programs, 2004. http://usinfo.state.gov.
4. Wikipedia. Expert witness. http://en.wikipedia.org/wiki/Expert_witness.
5. Preparing to testify. General resource guide. United States Department of Justice, United States attorney's office, Western District of Louisiana, 2010.
6. Daley, T.T. Guidelines for the expert witness. http://www.lectlaw.com/files/exp27.htm.
7. Kramer, I.R. and Connolly, J.M. Ten tips for testimony: Preparing for the witness stand. http://www.kramerslaw.com/evidence/testifying-tips.
8. M.K.G. Tips on the courtroom testimony. Get that extra edge over your opposition. http://www.internettradebureau.com/article/tips-on-courtroom-test.
9. Ashlock, S. Expert witness: Effective courtroom testimony. http://forensicmag.com/print/300
10. Murry, J. Sixteen tips on testing in court. http://pimall.com/nais/n.testify.html.
11. Hawkins, M.O. Introduction to courtroom testimony. http://hawkinspi.com/id27.html.

Alcohol Intoxication 13

In this chapter, several cases involving alcohol intoxication are presented. Drunk drivers take up considerable amount of time in hospital emergency rooms and toxicology laboratories, as well as with law enforcement personnel and the courts.

Alcoholism is a major problem in most countries in the world. Alcohol-induced traffic accidents are plentiful and sometimes have fatal outcomes. The loss of productivity at the workplace is considerable. Alcohol-related crimes take up considerable amount of time for law enforcement as well as the courts. For this reason, several countries enacted laws regarding legal limits of blood alcohol concentration (BAC) when operating motor vehicles. Laws regarding minimum age to operate a motor vehicle differ from country to country. In 1984, the United States enacted a national minimum drinking age. According to this law, a person must be 21 years of age to buy and drink alcoholic beverages. Again, these laws differ from country to country. To enforce drunken driving laws, law enforcement personnel need to measure BAC and relate it to intoxication and physiological performance of the operators. Thus far, blood is the preferred sample to measure alcohol levels. Urine and saliva as well as other body fluids have limited success.

Hospitals prefer using blood serum for measuring alcohol and for medical management of the patient, whereas law enforcement and the judiciary use BAC. Since punishment for driving under the influence (DUI) is based on BAC, serum alcohol levels need to be converted to blood alcohol levels. This is done by dividing by 1.1 to 1.18 (**1**).

Ethanol, ethyl alcohol, or what is commonly known as alcohol, is a water-soluble compound and is readily distributed into several body compartments including the brain. BAC reflects the alcohol reaching the brain and this in turn reflects the level of alcohol intoxication. BAC depends on the number of drinks consumed, their alcohol content, and the period in which they were consumed. BAC also depends upon the time lapse between the last drink and the time at which the BAC was measured. In addition, BAC depends on body weight, age, gender, health, and use of prescription or over-the-counter medications. It takes between 60 to 90 minutes for alcohol to be completely absorbed from the GI tract and reach peak levels in the blood. In some individuals, this is known to take more than 2 hours. Food in the stomach delays absorption. Alcohol is metabolized by the liver and is dissipated from the blood at a rate of 0.02% per hour (**1-6**).

13.1   Calculation of BAC

It is scientifically accepted that a 150-lb man will have a BAC of 0.025% after drinking 1 oz. of 100 proof (50%) alcohol. This assumption is accurate under almost all circumstances (**3**).

BAC= 150 ÷ Body weight × % ethanol content ÷ 50 × Ounces consumed × 0.025

A female has higher body fat and less body water than a man does. To be more rigorous, the above equation has to be multiplied by 1.17 or 1.2 to get the BAC of a female (**4,7**).

13.2   DUI, Hit-and-Run

13.2.1   Legal Aspects: DUI, Hit-and-Run, and Fatal Accident

This case is about the death of Joseph Gonzalez, a teenage cyclist who was hit by Susan Mulirala who was driving a car while intoxicated. The parents of Joseph brought a civil lawsuit against the bar for serving alcohol to Susan when she was intoxicated. They contend this caused the accident resulting in the untimely death of their teenage son and as such the bar should bear full responsibility for the accident. They demanded monetary compensation for their son's death. The bar owner said that Susan was a chronic alcoholic and did not show visible signs of intoxication.

13.2.2   Medical Aspects: Alcohol and Visible
Signs of Intoxication

The pharmacokinetics and metabolism of alcohol are well known. A correlation between blood alcohol levels, the intoxicating effects, and visible signs of intoxication are also very well known.

13.2.3   Factual Background

This report deals with a fatal accident on October 16, 2005, involving a car driven by Susan Mulirala, which hit Joseph Gonzalez, a cyclist, at 1:15 a.m. Joseph Gonzalez was a 15-year-old Caucasian male. Susan fled the scene and was later arrested by the police. She pleaded guilty and was incarcerated.

According to the police incident report, the accident happened in front of Kallu Lodge at 361 Yanam Road. Three teenage boys were riding their bicycles going eastbound on Yanam Road. Joseph Gonzalez was riding his yellow bicycle along with two of his teenage friends. A car also going east on Yanam Road at a high rate of speed hit Joseph Gonzalez from behind. The car did not apply the brakes and stop, but instead fled the scene. The ambulance was called in at 1:21 and arrived at the scene by 1:23 a.m. The police arrived at the scene and determined that the accident happened at 1:15 a.m. Autopsy revealed that Joseph died due to blunt impact trauma.

13.2.4   Events Leading up to the Accident

Police investigation revealed that a 2000 Toyota Corolla driven by Susan Mulirala hit Joseph. She is a 36-year-old Caucasian female, who weighed between 170 and 180 pounds on the day of the accident. She pleaded guilty for driving a motor vehicle while intoxicated. She also pleaded guilty for hitting Joseph Gonzalez, causing the fatal accident, and leaving the scene of the accident. According to the deposition testimony given by Susan Mulirala, she worked for South-Central Railways. She was divorced in 2000. On October 15, 2005, she went to work at 8:00 a.m. and left work at 4:00 p.m. She was at home by 5:15 p.m. She and her friend Josephine Border decided to meet at Vaneera Bar at 23 Luster Road. She was the first one to arrive at Vaneera Bar before Josephine and ordered a glass of wine around 6:30 p.m. Josephine arrived later and they sat at a bar table. Susan drank only white wine. Josephine drank Firewater. They also had a chicken dish and spinach dip. Susan's wine was served in a wine glass by bartenders. Each drink served to Susan was 6 oz. Susan and Josephine met two other male customers at the bar and were engaged in conversation with them. One of the male customers ordered a round of drinks for everyone at the bar around 8:15 p.m. Susan also met Patrick Lombardo at the bar. When he saw Susan, he recognized her and recalled that he met Susan a couple of times before at her job. They were having a good time discussing politics and having small talk. Susan says that Patrick also ordered drinks for her. Thus, according to the bar tabs, drinks were ordered and entered into accounts of each at various times, which provided the times at which the wine was served to Susan. Susan says she was sitting at the bar the entire time except when she went out to smoke cigarettes. She did not drink any wine before coming to the bar that evening. She also did not drink any other alcoholic beverage after she left the bar. Susan remembers that she came out of the bar and drove her car down Boulevard of the Rallis to Grand Street and made a left by a Toyota dealership. She then drove to Yanam Road and then to Elm Street. Suddenly she felt a jolt and did not know what she hit. She then drove to Chaps Bar at West Point. She did not remember how she got home. The next day, with the help of Josephine, she located her car parked near Chaps Bar. Her car had significant damage to the front end.

13.2.5 Blood Alcohol Concentration

BAC depends on several factors, which were listed previously (1-3). If the number of drinks consumed, their serving size, and the alcoholic content are known, it is possible to calculate the BAC of Susan at various time intervals. Based on these calculated values of BAC, it is easily possible to determine the level of intoxication of Susan.

It is scientifically accepted that a 150-lb man will have a BAC of 0.025% after drinking 1 oz. of 50% alcohol. Females have generally higher BAC than males of equal body weight due to differences in volume of distribution (Vd; volume/mass). A man is expected to have a Vd of 0.7 and a woman 0.6. These differences are due to differences in body water. In addition, a woman has less alcohol dehydrogenase enzyme activity than a man does, which metabolizes alcohol slower than a man. Therefore, a woman on average will have approximately 1.2 times more BAC when compared to a man of equal size (4,7).

$$\text{BAC (man)} = 150 \div \text{Body Wt.} \times \% \text{ ethanol content} \div 50 \times \text{ounces consumed} \times 0.025$$

$$\text{BAC (woman)} = 150 \div \text{Body Wt.} \times \% \text{ ethanol content} \div 50 \times \text{ounces consumed} \times 0.025 \times 1.17$$

It is assumed that Susan drank 6-oz. glasses of wine. Based on the bar tabs, it is possible to reconstruct the times at which the bartenders served wine to Susan. Wine has an alcoholic content of 12% (8). Susan's body weight at the time of the accident was 180 pounds. Based on these assumptions, her BAC at various times would be as follows (4):

$$\text{BAC} = 150 \div 180 \times 12 \div 50 \times 6 \times 0.025 \times 1.17 = 0.035$$

or, rounding to the second decimal place, it would be 0.04.

Only the number of drinks served to Susan according to bar tabs is taken into account in calculating Susan's BAC. Evidence by eyewitness testimony suggests that Susan probably had a drink at 6:30 p.m. when Josephine entered the bar. This was not on the bar tab. This drink was not considered. One additional round of drinks was purchased at approximately 8:15 p.m. by a male acquaintance. This is not recorded in the bar tab and hence not taken into account.

Calculated BAC of Susan Mulirala

Time (h)	Number of Drinks	Expected BAC (%)	Dissipated from Blood (%)	Calculated BAC (%)	Comments
6:30 p.m.		0	0	0	Entered bar
7:00 p.m.	1	0	0	0	
7:30 p.m.	2	0.04	0.01	0.03	
8:00 p.m.	3	0.08	0.02	0.06	
8:45 p.m.	4	0.12	0.035	0.085	
9:30 p.m.	5	0.16	0.05	0.11	
10:00 p.m.	6	0.20	0.06	0.14 (A)	
10:30 p.m.	7	0.24	0.07	0.17	
11:15 p.m.	8	0.28	0.085	0.195 (B)	
11:45 p.m.	0	0.32	0.095	0.225	
12:00 a.m.	0	0.32	0.10	0.22	
12:15 a.m.	0	0.32	0.105	0.215	Left bar (C)
1:15 a.m.	0	0.32	0.125	0.195	Accident (D)

13.2.6   BAC and Level of Intoxication

Susan admitted that she drank enough alcohol and got intoxicated. At approximately 10:00 p.m., she felt tipsy and things were fuzzy. She felt very much intoxicated and when she came back into the bar after smoking a cigarette, she could not walk straight. She does not remember the events after 10:00 p.m. She claims that somebody must have put GHB in her wine because it tasted different. In all probability, she left Vaneera Bar around 12:15 a.m.

According to Luke O'Maley, he walked to the bar and arrived there at approximately 7:00 p.m. He sat at the bar, there were plenty of seats, and the bar was not crowded. He drank cranberry juice. According to his statement to the police, Susan appeared drunk. He told police that he offered to get a cab for Susan and Josephine.

Susan went to Chaps Bar after the accident at 1:15 a.m. The bartender observed that she was drunk. She was staggering and fell off the chair two to three times. She wanted a drink, but the bartender refused to serve her. Instead, he gave her club soda. She was intoxicated at this point and needed help to get into a cab.

From the in-text table, it is obvious that Susan was expected to show the following signs and symptoms of alcohol intoxication:

A. At 10:03 p.m. the bartender served her a sixth drink, even though he knew that she had already consumed five drinks starting at 7:00 p.m. When she got this drink, her BAC was already 0.11%. Susan admitted that she was intoxicated and could not walk straight when

she entered the bar after smoking a cigarette. Susan started showing visual signs of intoxication. At this BAC, Susan was expected to
experience impairment of reaction responses, attention, visual acuity, sensory-motor coordination, and judgment. There was increased
drowsiness and emotional liability.

B. The bartender served Susan her seventh drink at 10:30 p.m. in spite
of Susan showing visual signs of intoxication. It is surprising that
the bartender served her an eighth drink at 11:15 p.m. This is her last
drink before she left the bar. At this point, her BAC was 0.195%. She
was expected to show visual signs/symptoms of intoxication such as
impairment of sensory-motor activities, reaction times, visual acuity, and judgment with progressive increase in drowsiness, disorientation, and emotional liability.

C. Susan left the bar at approximately 12:15 a.m. Her BAC was 0.215%
and she was showing signs and symptoms of intoxication. Still, the
bartender did not assist her and offer to get her a cab. According to
the statement given to police by Luke O'Maly, he offered to get Susan
a cab because she appeared drunk.

D. At the time of the accident at 1:15 a.m., Susan's BAC was 0.195%.
This accident was bound to happen as Susan experienced impairment of sensory-motor activities, reaction times, visual acuity, and
judgment. She probably experienced drowsiness and disorientation.
According to her testimony, she must have dozed off at the wheel.

When Susan entered Chaps Bar after the accident at 1:15 a.m., her BAC
probably was 0.195%. At this BAC, Susan showed visual signs of intoxication, which the bartender at Chaps Bar recognized and refused to serve her
alcoholic drinks.

Some chronic alcoholics develop tolerance and mask symptoms and signs
of alcohol intoxication. However, it is not possible to argue that Susan was
able to mask many signs and symptoms of alcohol intoxication at Vaneera
Bar for the following reasons:

- Susan testified that by 10:00 p.m. she was intoxicated and was
staggering.
- She was sitting at the bar in close proximity of the bartender and the
bar was not busy. There was no way the bartender could have missed
her visual signs of intoxication.
- When she was served one last drink at 11:15 p.m., her BAC was
0.195%. This increased to 0.215% when she left the bar. When she
entered Chaps Bar later, her BAC decreased to around 0.18 to 0.19%
as alcohol dissipated due to time lapse. At Chaps Bar they recognized
that Susan was intoxicated. The bartender refused to serve alcohol to

her. She was not able to walk and needed help to get into a cab. If the bartender at Chaps could recognize Susan was intoxicated and was not fit to drive her car, then the bartender at Vaneera Bar cannot say that Susan did not show visual signs of intoxication because her BAC was much higher at Vaneera Bar than at Chaps Bar.

13.2.7   Conclusions

Based on the available evidence, it can be concluded with a reasonable degree of medical and scientific certainty that:

1. Susan Mulirala was sitting at the bar and was served seven glasses of wine in approximately 6 hours at Vaneera Bar by the bartenders.
2. Susan did show visual signs and symptoms of alcohol intoxication both at Vaneera and at Chaps. At Chaps, they refused to serve alcohol to Susan and put her in a cab and sent her home, whereas at Vaneera, they continued to serve her alcohol and did not offer to get her a cab.
3. The bartenders at Vaneera were irresponsible in not refusing to serve alcohol to Susan when she was intoxicated. Susan was in no condition to drive.
4. Vaneera Bar was more concerned about liquor sales, which resulted in Susan being intoxicated prior to the fatal accident. Thus, Vaneera Bar is responsible for the untimely and unnecessary death of Joseph Gonzalez.

13.3   DUI, Auto Accident, Death of Passenger

13.3.1   Legal Aspects: Fatal Accident Due to Alcohol Intoxication

Debbie Gillichi is suing David Binder for the accidental death of her husband John Gillichi, who was a passenger in a Cadillac Deville driven by David Binder. In this civil suit, Debbie is demanding monetary compensation. She further contends that her husband and David were together, that David was intoxicated with alcohol and possibly cocaine, and was thus unfit to drive a motor vehicle.

13.3.2   Medical Aspects

David Binder's BAC was above the legal limit (0.1%). Unfortunately, no drug screens were performed on his blood or urine. Therefore, it is not possible to know the effects of other drugs in his blood in addition to the very high alcohol levels in his blood at the time of the accident. He was intoxicated, lost control of the car, and caused a fatal accident that resulted in the death of John Gillichi.

13.3.3 Factual Background

David Binder is a 45-year-old white male, 5 feet 8 inches tall, weighing 165 pounds. The passenger was John Gillichi, a 47-year-old white male, 6 feet 2 inches tall, weighing 250 pounds. David was driving a 1992 Cadillac Deville on April 18, 1999. He lost control of the car, crossed onto the opposite lane, and entered a ditch. The car rolled over several times. John, the passenger, was thrown out of the car and sustained multiple fractures and serious injuries resulting in his death at the scene. David was bleeding and starting walking. He was found by witnesses walking on the road to get help. According to police, the accident happened at 4:05 a.m. The police arrived at the scene and found David bleeding and smelling of alcohol. The police contend that the preliminary breath test (PBT) breathalyzer test gave a BAC of 0.155% at 5:15 a.m. His blood was drawn at a local hospital and was analyzed at Michigan State Forensic Laboratory, which gave a BAC of 0.14%.

It appears that John and David were together at a bar and stayed there until 2:00 a.m. They then went to Camp at Half Moon Bay. They played cards and had a few more drinks. They left the camp and were driving home on CR 550 at 65 mph. David lost control of the car at 4:05 a.m. Unfortunately, the police requested that David's blood be tested for alcohol. Instead, they should have requested an analysis of his blood and urine for drugs as well. The passenger's body fluids at autopsy showed presumptive presence of cocaine and its metabolite. A complete autopsy of the body of the deceased was not conducted and consequently no such report is available. The pathologist, John D. Martinez, MD, conducted only an external examination and obtained urine, blood, and vitreous fluid. These were sent for toxicology analysis to AST Laboratories, Scranton, Pennsylvania. The report by the pathologist showed that the deceased suffered multiple fractures to the chest and face, and lacerations on other parts of the body with blood exuding from the nose and mouth. The toxicology report showed that blood contained 0.112% ethanol, less than 50 ng/ml of cocaine, and less than 50 ng/ml of benzoylecogonine. No other drugs were found in the blood or urine. The pathologist did not interpret the toxicology results. Dr. Ellis of AST Laboratories said that drugs of abuse in blood and urine were screened by immunoassay and confirmed by GC-MS. In addition, drugs of abuse in the blood were also quantitated by GC-MS.

13.3.4 Blood Alcohol Concentration

Blood alcohol levels depend on several factors as listed previously (1-3). David's BAC was above the legal limit (0.08%). Unfortunately, no drug screens were performed on blood or urine of David. Therefore, we do not know the effect of other substances in his blood in addition to the very high alcohol levels at the time of the accident. It is no wonder he lost control of the car and caused a fatal accident (1-3). The deceased suffered multiple fractures and his chest was crushed. Under these conditions, the blood was likely to be contaminated with his stomach contents. His blood alcohol levels at 0.112% appear to be true as these BAC closely correlate with vitreous fluid alcohol levels at 0.122% (1). The BAC of the deceased reiterates that David and John were drinking. The BAC of the deceased has no contribution to the accident because he was only a passenger.

13.3.5 Cocaine and Its Metabolites in Blood and Urine

Cocaine is one of the most potent drugs that stimulate the central nervous system. Cocaine abuse is considerable in this country. Intake of cocaine is through several routes of administration. These include inhalation of cocaine smoke, injection, snorting, and dermal application. Whatever may be the route of administration, cocaine is absorbed rapidly and appears in the blood in approximately 10 minutes. The half-life of cocaine in blood is approximately 30 to 40 minutes and it disappears from the blood within 6 to 8 hours. Immediately after absorption, cocaine is metabolized to benzoylec-gonine, which starts appearing in the blood 10 to 15 minutes after ingesting cocaine. Cocaine metabolites can be detected in urine up to 72 hours after use. A single dose of cocaine is expected to give a peak plasma concentration between 200 ng/ml and 400 ng/ml. The presence of cocaine and its metabo-lites in blood and urine are detected by immunoassay and is generally con-firmed by GC-MS. According to NIDA, the cutoff value for immunoassay is 300 ng/ml and for GC-MS, it is 150 ng/ml (11). Even though no such cutoff values apply to an autopsy sample, it is possible to conclude that the values below the cutoff may be due to secondhand or unintentional intake (5,6). The toxicology report by AST Laboratories shows low levels of cocaine and benzoylecgonine in the blood of the deceased. Given the short half-life of cocaine, it is reasonable to argue that the deceased was exposed to cocaine immediately before he got in the car with David. Cocaine in urine was not quantitated but was positive, suggesting that these levels were also below the cutoff values for GC-MS. Environmental exposure to cocaine is a real possi-bility and can occur through unintentional skin contact or due to side stream exposure to cocaine smoke (9,10).

If the deceased indeed abused cocaine prior to the accident, his blood levels of cocaine or its metabolite should have been at least 200 to 400 ng/ml. However, the results were below 50 ng/ml; this could be anywhere between 0 and 50 ng/ml. That is why NIDA does not consider these extremely low values as evidence of drug abuse (11). These results only prove that the deceased was in a place where cocaine was used. Even though the deceased cannot defend himself, it is the responsibility of the toxicologist to recognize that extreme caution is warranted when interpreting low levels of cocaine or cocaine metabolite in blood and urine. Skin contact unintentionally can result in urinary benzoylecgonine levels. Similarly, sidestream smoke exposure to cocaine can cause considerable quantities of cocaine and cocaine metabolites in blood and urine. That is why NIDA established 150 ng/ml and 300 ng/ml cutoff values for GC-MS and immunoassay, respectively (**3,9**).

13.3.6   Conclusions

It can be concluded with a reasonable degree of scientific certainty that:

1. David Binder and John Gillichi were at a place where cocaine was used.
2. David did consume a considerable amount of alcoholic beverages but it is not possible to draw conclusions on his cocaine use as no drug screens were performed.
3. John probably did not intentionally take cocaine but was exposed to accidental skin contact or side-stream cocaine smoke.
4. Results that were below the cutoff levels for cocaine and its metabolite in blood and urine support the above contention.

13.4   DUI, Automobile Accident, Death of a Passenger

13.4.1   Legal Aspects: DUI, Death of a Passenger

A fatal car accident happened on July 29, 2001 at approximately 10:10 p.m. James Kisko, a 19-year-old white male was the driver of a white Toyota Corolla and the passenger was a 20-year-old white male, Richard Simmons. James was driving without valid automobile insurance. They were coming home after attending a marriage reception in Jennet Township. James lost control of the car and went off the road. His car hit the trees, rolled over, and landed on its roof. James had minor injuries while Richard died at the scene due to his severe injuries. Mrs. Simmons, the mother of the deceased, sued the fathers of the bride and the groom for unrestricted access to beer at the reception, which she alleges caused the accident resulting in her son's death. She demands financial compensation for wrongful death of her son. The defendants contend that they are not responsible because Richard got into the car of his own free will and should have realized that James was too intoxicated to drive.

13.4.2 Medical Aspects: Alcohol Intoxication

James and Richard reached the wedding reception at approximately 4:00 p.m. and drank beer for the next 5 hours. They left the wedding reception at approximately 9:00 p.m. They were intoxicated. They got into the car and proceeded to go home on highway SR 65. After the accident, police brought James to the hospital where his blood was drawn at 12:30 a.m. His BAC was 0.11%. Toxicology analysis of Richard's blood taken at autopsy gave a BAC of 0.25%. James's BAC suggests that he was intoxicated and was unfit to drive.

13.4.3 Factual Background

This report deals with a fatal car accident that occurred on July 29, 2001 at approximately at 10:10 p.m. James Kisko, a 19-year-old white male, was the driver of a white Toyota Corolla and the passenger Richard Simmons, a 20-year-old white male. The car was coming from the town of Jennet and was going home on SR 65. James's blood was drawn at 12:30 a.m. and a blood alcohol test was done at the hospital, which gave a BAC of 0.11%. James and Richard were going home after attending a marriage reception in Jennet. James lost control of the car, which went off the road, hit trees, rolled over, and landed on its roof. The road was wet in places with intermittent fog. Both the driver and the passenger were not wearing seat belts. The passenger was thrown out of the car and landed by the side of the car. Both the driver and the passenger sustained injuries. The passenger received multiple traumas and died at the scene.

James left the scene after obtaining a ride to his home apparently to get help. On reaching his home, he called 911. The paramedics came to James's home. James was transported to the Community Hospital in Peter's Township. Richard was pronounced dead by the coroner at 12:18 a.m. on July 30, 2001. Richard's body was also taken to Community Hospital.

James and Richard were friends and attended the same high school. Richard's brother dropped him off at James Kisko's house. They then proceeded to Jannet to attend a wedding reception. They reached the wedding reception at approximately 4:00 p.m. They had unrestricted access to beer and they drank for the next 5 hours. They left the wedding reception at approximately 9:00 p.m.

The police arrived at the accident site at 11:50 p.m. Based on police interviews with several people, the time of the accident was estimated to be 10:10 p.m. The police went to Community Hospital and interviewed James at 1:35 a.m. The police officer noticed a strong smell of alcohol coming from James. James's blood was drawn at 12:30 a.m. and a blood alcohol test was done at the hospital laboratory. It showed a BAC of 0.11%. The autopsy on the body of Richard was conducted on July 30, 2001. The autopsy indicated blunt force trauma to the abdomen and chest, and multiple lacerations to several organs. Toxicology analysis of Richard's blood taken at autopsy gave a BAC of 0.25%.

13.4.4   Blood Alcohol Concentration

BAC depends on several factors as listed previously (1,2,9). Here the BAC of the two involved individuals can be worked out as follows.

13.4.4.1   James Kisko

James left the reception at 9:00 p.m. after his last drink. The accident happened at 10:10 p.m. and his blood was drawn at the hospital at 12:30 a.m., approximately 3.5 hours after his last drink. His BAC was determined to be 0.11. His calculated BAC at various time intervals after he left the reception area, would be as follows:

Time (h)	BAC (%)	Comments
9:00 p.m.	0.18	Left the reception
9:30 p.m.	0.17	
10:00 p.m.	0.16	
10:10 p.m.	0.156	Accident
10:30 p.m.	0.15	
11:00 p.m.	0.14	
11:30 p.m.	0.13	
12:00 a.m.	0.12	
12:30 a.m.	0.11	Blood draw

His estimated BAC when he left the reception area would be 0.18% and at the time of the accident, his BAC would be 0.156%. At this BAC, a person exhibits impairment of motor skills and coordination, loss of balance, loss of visual acuity, and drowsiness (4).

13.4.4.2   Richard Simmons

Richard left the reception area with James at 9:00 p.m. He probably died after the accident at approximately 11:00 p.m. His autopsy BAC showed 0.25%. His calculated BAC at various times would be as follows:

Time (h)	BAC (%)	Comments
9:00 p.m.	0.29	Left reception
9:30 p.m.	0.28	
10:00 p.m.	0.27	
10:10 p.m.	0.266	Accident
10:30 p.m.	0.26	
11:00 p.m.	0.25	Death

Richard Simmons's BAC at the time he left the reception area would be 0.29%. At this BAC, he would be expected to show disorientation, mental confusion, dizziness, loss of critical judgment, loss of motor coordination, staggering, apathy, sleep, or stupor (4). In other words, Richard was intoxicated three times the legal limit and was not aware of his surroundings.

13.4.5 Conclusions

1. Richard was highly intoxicated and was not aware of his surroundings when he left the reception area and got into the car driven by James.
2. Clearly, Richard's behavior was consistent with the level of his intoxication. He lost his critical judgment, as he was in a stupor and was sleepy, disoriented, and confused.
3. Therefore, he was not in a position to judge the danger he was putting himself into by getting into a car driven by James.
4. James was intoxicated and his BAC was close to two times the legal limit when he left the reception area and started driving the car.
5. James's BAC was 0.156% at the time of the accident. He was intoxicated and clearly unfit to drive.

13.5 DUI, Death of a Motorcyclist

13.5.1 Legal Aspects: Presumptive DUI and Motorcycle Accident

Michael Skipper was driving his Jeep with his friend as his passenger. A motorcyclist coming at a great rate of speed in the same direction crashed onto the Jeep when Michael was taking a left turn onto the driveway of his house. The motorcyclist died a few days later at the hospital. The police administered a PBT test and charged Michael with DUI and vehicular homicide.

13.5.2 Medical Aspects: BAC and Alcohol Intoxication

Correlation between BAC and alcohol levels reaching the brain and the resulting alcohol intoxication are well established. Therefore, it is important to correlate the blood alcohol levels at the time of the accident with the alcohol levels at the time of the blood draw. Otherwise, the driver of the Jeep would be charged with vehicular homicide even though he was not intoxicated.

13.5.3 Factual Background

Michael Skipper is an African American male, 28 years of age, 5 feet 10 inches tall, and weighing 165 pounds on June 11, 2000, the day of the accident. The defendant was driving a Jeep north on Pine Road and was making a left turn onto his driveway on 343 Pine Road after using his left turn signal. The motorcycle driven by Chuck Williams was also going north on Pine Road at 75 mph on a 35 mph road. He overtook several cars and crashed into the driver's side of the Jeep, which was driven by the defendant. The accident happened at approximately 1:40 a.m. Both drivers sustained injuries and Chuck subsequently died at St. Bervenuti Hospital due to the injuries sustained in the collision.

According to the account given to the police, the defendant left his house at 9:30 p.m. the previous evening, arrived at Sachee's Road House, and remained there until 11:20 p.m. He ate his dinner and did not drink any alcoholic beverages during his dinner. He left Sachee's Road House and arrived at High-Ho Bar at 11:30 p.m. He had three beers and a large shot of tequila before he left the bar. He picked up a friend who was a passenger in the car at the time of the accident at 1:40 a.m.

The police arrived at the scene at approximately 2:15 a.m. The police officer interviewed several witnesses including the defendant. The police officer administered a PBT test to the defendant at approximately 2:30 a.m., which gave a reading of 0.1% BAC. The defendant was charged with DUI and taken to a community hospital, where his blood was drawn at 3:30 a.m. and was analyzed by GC by the county police laboratory. This analysis gave a BAC of 0.17%. Since GC determination of BAC is a gold standard and analytical procedures by the laboratory appear to be proper, there were no grounds to challenge this result. Unfortunately, the hospital did not analyze the blood of Chuck Williams before he died.

13.5.4 Blood Alcohol Concentration

BAC depends on several factors as listed previously (1,2,4,5). The defendant ate a heavy meal at Sachee's Road House and ate snacks while drinking at the High-Ho Bar.

The defendant's last drink at the bar was at 1:30 a.m. He left the bar at 1:35 a.m., and the accident happened at 1:40 a.m. The police arrived at the scene at 2:15 a.m. The PBT test was administered to the defendant at approximately 2:30 a.m., which gave a BAC of 0.1%. This was 1 hour prior to the blood draw at 3:30 a.m., for alcohol analysis by a GC, which gave a BAC of 0.17%. Therefore, the defendant was in the absorptive stage of alcohol metabolism. Given this fact, it is possible to calculate the defendant's BAC at various times including the time at which the accident took place. Since there is a time lapse of 2 h between the defendant's last drink and the time of the blood draw, the defendant was expected to dissipate at least 0.03% of alcohol from his blood. Therefore, this needs to be added to 0.175, which gives a calculated BAC of 0.20% at 3:30 a.m. Therefore, the calculated BAC at various time intervals would be as follows:

Time (h)	BAC (%)	Comments
1:30 a.m.	0	Last drink
1:35 a.m.	0	Left the bar
1:40 a.m.	0	Accident
1:45 a.m.	0.025	
2:00 a.m.	0.05	
2:15 a.m.	0.075	
2:30 a.m.	0.10	PBT Test
2:45 a.m.	0.103	
3:00 a.m.	0.150	
3:15 a.m.	0.175	
3:30 a.m.	0.20	Blood draw

From the previously calculated BAC, it can easily be inferred that the defendant's BAC at the time of the accident should be between 0 and 0.025%. The BAC of 0.17% in the blood drawn at 3:30 only proves the BAC at this time but not at the time of the accident. For this reason, the defendant should not be penalized by improper interpretation of his BAC. The accident happened through no fault of the defendant. The motorcyclist may have been intoxicated because he was going at a great rate of speed, overtaking several vehicles before crashing into the Jeep, which was making a left turn to enter the driveway of the defendant's house.

13.5.5   Conclusions

It can be concluded with a reasonable degree of scientific certainty that:

1. The defendant's BAC at the time of the accident was between 0 and 0.025%.
2. The PBT test taken at 2:30 a.m. gave a BAC of 0.1%. The BAC determined in the blood sample drawn at 3:30 a.m. gave a reading of 0.17%.
3. These results support the contention that the defendant was in the absorptive phase of alcohol metabolism.
4. The calculation of BAC at various intervals suggests that BAC at the time of accident was so low that alcohol intoxication of the defendant had no role in this unfortunate accident.

13.6   DUI, Hit-and-Run

13.6.1   Legal Aspects: DUI, Hit-and-Run

Jennifer Dessi was driving a rental car from the airport on Route 50 going toward downtown Plottsburgh, Pennsylvania. She was intoxicated with alcohol. The traffic was heavy on the highway. She hit a car in front of her, which in turn bumped a car in front of it. Jennifer suddenly took off and went to her ex-husband's house. The police caught up with her and arrested her for presumptive DUI. She contends that she drank three glasses of wine at her ex-husband's house after the accident and therefore she was not intoxicated at the time of the accident.

13.6.2   Medical Aspects: Alcohol Metabolism

The pharmacokinetics and metabolism of alcohol are well known. Even though the defendant drank alcohol at her ex-husband's house, it is still possible to calculate and establish her BAC at the time of accident.

13.6.3   Factual Background

This case involves a hit-and-run accident on July 24, 2004 at 9:30 p.m. The accident involved three cars, all traveling east on Route 50 near Plottsburgh, Pennsylvania.

Jennifer Dessi is a Caucasian female, 46 years of age, 5 feet 7 inches tall, and weighing 150 pounds on the day of the accident. She was employed as a flight attendant by Queens Airlines and lives at 9275 Skyward Road, Plottsburgh, Pennsylvania. On the day of the accident, Jennifer claims she consumed two 5-oz. glasses of red wine at her friend's house between 7:15 p.m. and 8:15 p.m. She does not recall the brand of wine.

The car that Jennifer hit contained Erin Raws, who was driving, and Beverly Bisek.

The traffic on Route 50 was heavy. When they were near Sandow Corporation, the car driven by Jennifer hit the plaintiffs' car, resulting in the plaintiffs' car hitting the car in front of them.

At the scene, Erin and Beverly observed that Jennifer smelled of alcohol, and they both believed her to be drunk. They observed bloodshot and watery eyes, saw Jennifer fumbling about, and observed that she was not answering questions, appeared to be confused, had a hard time focusing, and was belligerent. Jennifer pleaded with the plaintiffs not to call the police. When Beverly was on her cell phone reporting the accident to the police, Jennifer suddenly went to the shoulder of the road and drove away from the scene.

Jennifer says that she left the scene of the accident and drove to her ex-husband's house where she consumed three glasses of wine. She claims she does not recall the brand of wine. She then went to her own house where the police arrived and apprehended her at approximately 12:00 a.m. The police observed that Jennifer was visibly intoxicated. An initial breathalyzer test suggested that she was drunk. The police then took her to the police station and administered a breath alcohol test using the Intoxilyzer 5000 at 12:24 a.m. This breathalyzer test revealed a BAC of 0.17%. The police charged Jennifer with driving under the influence and leaving the scene of an accident. She subsequently pled guilty for driving under the influence and was accepted into the ARD (Accelerated Rehabilitative Disposition) program for first-time offenders.

The accident resulted in damage to the rental car driven by the plaintiffs. Beverly sustained serious injuries to the neck and back area. She had to undergo physical rehabilitation and chiropractic treatments. Erin sustained injuries to her neck and back area.

13.6.4 Blood Alcohol Concentration

BAC depends on several factors as stated previously. For a normal healthy male weighing 200 pounds, one alcoholic drink gives a BAC of 0.02%. The same individual also dissipates 0.02% alcohol from the blood in 1 hour (1,2,4,5).

It is scientifically accepted that a 150-lb man will have a BAC of 0.025% after drinking 1 oz. of 50% alcohol (3). The formula is expressed as follows:

$$BAC = 150 \div \text{Body weight} \times \% \text{ ethanol content} \div 50 \times \text{ounces consumed} \times 0.025$$

A female has higher body fat and less body water than a man does. To be more rigorous, the above equation has to be multiplied by 1.2 to get the BAC of a female (7). Therefore, for a female, the following is true:

$$BAC = 150 \div \text{Body weight} \times \% \text{ ethanol content} \div 50 \times \text{ounces consumed} \times 0.025 \times 1.2$$

Jennifer Dessi's body weight is taken as 150 pounds at the time of the accident.

She claims she does not recall the brand of wine she consumed. The alcoholic content of wine can vary between 8 and 14% (12). An average is 11%. It is assumed that the wine she consumed had 11% alcoholic content.

The BAC of Jennifer after consuming a 5-oz. glass of 11% wine is calculated as follows:

$$BAC = 150 \div 150 \times 11 \div 50 \times 5 \times 0.025 \times 1.2 = 0.03\%$$

Jennifer's BAC was determined to be 0.17% at 12:24 a.m. Yet, she contends that she drank three more glasses of wine after the accident at her ex-husband's house. Assuming this is true (and there is no support for this in the record other than Jennifer's own testimony), the BAC of 0.096% contributed by three additional glasses of wine is subtracted from the BAC of 0.17%. This leaves a BAC of .074%.

It is expected that alcohol would be absorbed completely in approximately 30 minutes. Alcohol is dissipated from the blood at the rate of 0.02% in 1 hour. The dissipation of alcohol from the blood at the rate of 0.02% per hour is used to back calculate Jennifer's BAC at various times as follows:

Time (h)	BAC (%)	Dissipation (%)	Calculated BAC	Comments
9:00 p.m.		0.07	0.144	Left friend's house
9:30 p.m.		0.06	0.134	Accident
10:00 p.m.		0.05	0.124	
10:30 p.m.		0.04	0.114	
11:00 p.m.		0.03	0.104	
11:30 p.m.		0.02	0.094	
12:00 a.m.		0.01	0.084	
12:24 a.m.	0.17–0.096	0.074	0	0.74 – Breathalyzer test

Based on these calculations, one can conclude that Jennifer consumed between three and four glasses of wine at her friend's house before the accident.

13.6.4.1 Alcohol Intoxication of Jennifer Dessi

Alcohol is a water-soluble compound, and reaches peak blood levels once it is absorbed from the GI tract and then distributed into body compartments. The pharmacology of alcohol and its toxic kinetics are well known. There is a perfect correlation between the BAC and the alcohol levels reaching the brain and their effect on the CNS and impairment of physiological functions (1).

Between 0.07 and 0.1% BAC, alcohol causes impairment of reaction times, judgment, attention, sensory motor coordination, and visual acuity.

Between 0.1 and 0.2% BAC, alcohol causes further intoxicating effects. In addition to the CNS effects mentioned previously, there is a progressive increase in drowsiness, disorientation, and emotional liability.

At a BAC of 0.1 to 0.2%, Jennifer is expected to feel the effects of intoxication such as drowsiness, staggering, impairment, and disorientation. She also would have loss of coordination, visual acuity, and judgment.

13.6.5 Conclusions

The case of Jennifer Dessi demonstrates a correlation between BAC and the effects of alcohol intoxication. At the time of the crash, her BAC was 0.134%. This suggests that alcohol intoxication impaired her judgment and slowed her reaction times. The fact that she rear-ended the plaintiffs' car with force confirms that alcohol impaired her visual acuity. Jennifer's BAC was above the legal limit at the time of the accident and all evidence indicates that she was drunk and unfit to drive.

It can be concluded with a reasonable degree of scientific certainty that:

1. At the time of the accident, Jennifer Dessi was drunk and her BAC was above the legal limit.
2. Jennifer Dessi was unfit to drive at the time of the accident.

13.7 DUI and a Two-Car Collision

13.7.1 Legal Aspects: Presumptive DUI and Motor Vehicle Accident

This case is about a motor vehicle accident on November 4, 2000 at 10:05 p.m. It is alleged in the police complaint that the defendant, Maggie Lederer, failed to stop at a stop sign and her Hyundai SUV hit a car driven by Peter Magoo. Both cars were damaged and were towed to Skip's Auto Service. Maggie was arrested for presumptive DUI. Maggie contests her arrest by the police and says her BAC must be below the legal limit at the time of the accident. The following two questions need to be answered by the prosecution:

1. Was the defendant in the absorptive phase of alcohol metabolism?
2. Was the defendant's BAC above the legal limit at the time of the accident?

13.7.2 Medical Aspects: Pre- and Post-Absorptive BAC

If the defendant was in the absorption phase of alcohol metabolism, her blood alcohol levels might be low and different from the blood alcohol levels seen at the time of her blood draw. Therefore, the defendant's BAC could be below the legal limit at the time of the accident.

13.7.3 Factual Background

This case is about a motor vehicle accident on November 4, 2000 at 10:05 p.m. The accident happened in Cactus Township at the intersection of Lawrence Avenue and Betalnut Street. It is alleged that the defendant, Maggie Lederer, failed to stop at a stop sign and her Hyundai SUV hit a car driven by Peter Magoo. Both cars were damaged and were towed to Skip's Auto Service. Maggie was driving north on Lawrence Avenue with three passengers at the time of the accident. The defendant is a Caucasian female, approximately 185 pounds, 5 feet 3 inches tall, and 39 years of age at the time of the accident. The defendant contends that she drank two beers between 2:00 p.m. and 3:00 p.m. She went to Redwood Volunteer Fireman's Club at 8:45 p.m. and drank three beers. She left the Fireman's club at 9:50 p.m. and proceeded to go to Dengle, Pennsylvania with her three passengers. Based on her responses to questions written by a toxicologist hired by the District Attorney, it was evident that she was a chronic alcoholic and used to drink until she passed out. She now contends that she has been sober since March 5, 2000. The accident scene is only 5 minutes away from the Fireman's Club.

When the police arrived, the defendant was standing outside her car near the front driver-side door. The passenger in the back seat appeared intoxicated. The front-seat passenger fled the scene but later appeared in court and stated that she was injured and was treated at a hospital. Even though the defendant failed sobriety tests, the police found that she had a moderate but not strong smell of alcohol on her breath. Her speech was fair but she was not stuttering, incoherent, or confused. She was arrested for presumptive DUI at 10:27 p.m., taken to Queens Area Hospital, and her blood was drawn at 11:11 p.m. Her blood analysis by the state police laboratory gave a BAC of 0.12%.

13.7.4   Blood Alcohol Concentration

BAC depends on several factors (1,2,4,5). The defendant weighed 185 pounds. Even though a female metabolizes alcohol at a slower rate than a man does, approximately one alcoholic drink is expected to give a BAC of 0.022%. She admits drinking two beers between 2:00 p.m. and 3:00 p.m. These two beers would have given her a BAC of 0.044%. She entered Fireman's Club at approximately 8:45 p.m. In those six hours, she was expected to dissipate all the alcohol from her blood. Given the number of beers she admits she drank at the Fireman's Club and the time of her accident, it is possible to calculate her BAC at various time intervals. Alcohol is rapidly absorbed from the GI tract and goes to the blood in approximately 60 to 90 minutes. However, in some individuals this absorption may not be complete even up to 2 hours after the last drink (1,2,4,5).

As stated earlier, two central questions need to be addressed to come to a reasonable conclusion regarding the level of intoxication by the defendant. These questions are:

1. Was the defendant in the absorptive phase of alcohol metabolism?
2. Was the defendant above the legal limit at the time of the accident?

Since there was a time lapse of 1 hour 21 minutes to the time at which her blood was drawn, she was expected to dissipate 0.03% of alcohol from her blood. This needs to be added to her BAC of 0.12% at her blood draw to arrive at her estimated BAC at 11:11 p.m. Her BAC is calculated as shown in the following table.

Time (h)	BAC (%)	Comments
9:50 p.m.	0	Left Fireman's Club
10:00 p.m.	0.01	
10:05 p.m.	0.02	Accident
10:10 p.m.	0.03	
10:20 p.m.	0.05	
10:30 p.m.	0.07	
10:40 p.m.	0.09	
10:50 p.m.	0.11	
11:00 p.m.	0.13	
11:11 p.m.	0.15	Blood draw

The table shows that her BAC at the time of the accident was approximately 0.02%. The fact that the police found her alcoholic breath to be moderate but not strong and her speech was fair but not incoherent or stuttering underscores that her BAC at the time of the accident was much below the legal limit.

13.7.5 Conclusions

Based on the evidence, it can be concluded with a reasonable degree of scientific certainty that:

1. The defendant was in an absorptive phase of alcohol metabolism.
2. Her BAC at the time of the accident was much below the legal limit.
3. BAC at the time of accident was so low that alcohol intoxication played no role in the accident.

References

1. DiMaio, V. J. and DiMaio, D. *Forensic Pathology*, 2nd ed. CRC Press, Boca Raton, FL, 2001.
2. Levine, B. *Principles of Forensic Toxicology*. AACC Press, Washington, D.C., 1999.
3. Karch, S.B. *Karch's Pathology of Drug Abuse*, 3rd ed. CRC Press, Boca Raton, FL, 2001.
4. Zernig, G., Saria, A., Kurz, M., and O'Malley, S.S., Eds. *Handbook of Alcoholism*. CRC Press, Boca Raton, FL, 2000.
5. Nakaya, A.C. *Alcoholism*. Greenhaven Press, Detroit, MI, 2008.

Forensic Toxicology: Medico-Legal Case Studies

6. Alcohol and the human body. http://www.padui.org/information/effects-of-drugs-and-alcohol.
7. Baraona, E., Abittan, C.S., Dohmen, K., Moretti, M., Pozatto, B., Chayes, Z.W., Schfer, C., and Lieber, C.S. Gender differences in pharmacokinetics of alcohol. *Alcoholism.* **25**:502–507, 2001.
8. Pinot Grigio. The Inimitables. www.santamargherita.com/prodetti_e/inimitabili/us/wine/pinot-grigio.
9. Isenshmid, D.S. Cocaine. In: *Principles of Forensic Toxicology*, Levine, B., Ed. American Association for Clinical Chemistry, Inc., Washington, D.C., 1999, 221–245.
10. Baselt, R.C. and Cravey, R.H. Disposition of Toxic Drugs and Chemicals in Man. Chemical Toxicology Institute, Foster City, CA, 1995, 186–190.
11. Casarett, L.J., Doull, J., and Klaasen, C.D. Casarett and Doull's toxicology: The basic science of poisons. *Federal Register* 53(69), 11983, 1988.
12. Alcohol content of some common drinks. alcoholcontents.com.

False-Positive Blood Alcohol

14

This chapter deals with several cases of false-positive blood alcohol levels. This can be due to analytical errors, interference from medication that the defendant was taking, or in the case of autopsy, the chest cavity may be contaminated by unabsorbed alcohol present in the stomach.

The enzymatic method of serum ethanol determination with alcohol dehydrogenase and NAD gave false-positive serum ethanol levels. The reason for this anomalous result of alcohol determination is given in detail in Chapter 3. To recap the principle of enzymatic alcohol determination, it can be seen that the automated analyzers utilize the following reaction:

$$\text{Ethylalcohol} + \text{NAD} \xrightarrow{\text{ADH}} \text{Acetaldehyde} + \text{NADH}$$

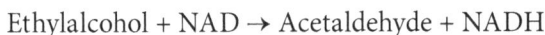

ADH = alcoholdehydrogenase; NAD = nicotinamide adenine dinucleotide

However, it became evident that the following reaction interferes and generates falsely elevated serum alcohol levels.

$$\text{Lactate} + \text{NAD} \xrightarrow{\text{LDH}} \text{Pyruvate} + \text{NADH}$$

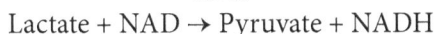

LDH = Lactate dehydrogenase

These enzymatic methods are rapid, quick, and cheaper. Again, as stated in Chapter 3, determination of alcohol by GC is the gold standard. Forensic laboratories and police toxicology laboratories use GC for ethanol determinations. In cases of automobile accidents involving severe trauma, both lactate and LDH increase and the elevated lactate does not clear rapidly (1,3-5). For this reason, a toxicologist needs to ascertain the method by which serum alcohol levels are measured.

False-positives can happen due to interference from a drug that competes with alcohol during metabolism by the liver.

False-positives may also occur during autopsy. In this case, the chest cavity blood may be contaminated with alcohol present in the stomach. In this case, the blood needs to be obtained from an alternative site and alcohol levels need to be checked in vitreous fluid (6).

14.1 Presumptive DUI, Two-Car Collision, Doctor's Death

14.1.1 Legal Aspects: Wrongful Death

This case is about a doctor's widow who brought a civil suit against the state of Arizona. The widow sought monetary compensation for the death of her husband who she believes died because of the state's negligence in failing to repair a state highway. She alleged that a Jeep driven by a teenager, Ricardo, with two other teenage passengers, lost control, entered the opposite lane, and collided head-on with the car driven by her husband. This accident happened on the state highway AR 83 at 7:45 p.m. On the other hand, the state of Arizona contends that Ricardo lost control of the Jeep he was driving because he was intoxicated.

14.1.2 Medical Aspects

The teenage driver of the Jeep survived but suffered multiple fractures and traumas. He was transferred to Jefferson Medical Center by helicopter at approximately 8:50 p.m. The emergency room obtained his blood at 9:46 p.m. and sent it to the laboratory for toxicology analysis. The laboratory reported serum alcohol level of 162 mg/dL or 0.162%.

14.1.3 Factual Background

The doctor was driving his car home after work northbound on AR 83. At the same time, a Jeep driven by a teenager and two other teenage passengers was coming in the opposite direction, lost control, entered the opposite lane, and collided head-on with the oncoming car. The teenage driver of the Jeep, Ricardo, survived but suffered multiple fractures and traumas. Two other teenage passengers in the Jeep and the doctor driving in the other car died at the accident scene.

Ricardo is a Caucasian male, 15 years of age, and weighing 115 pounds on the day of the accident. He was transferred to Jefferson Medical Center by a helicopter at approximately 8:50 p.m. He was admitted to the emergency room with multiple fractures, head injury, shock, and coma. The patient underwent surgical procedures and was discharged after three weeks.

Since the patient was hypotensive, he received a total of 3 L of Lactated Ringer's solution en route to the hospital. A few minutes after completion of the infusion of Lactated Ringer's solution, the emergency room obtained his blood at 9:46 p.m. and sent it to the laboratory for alcohol determination. The laboratory analysis reveals several-fold elevations of liver enzymes including LDH in serum. This is not surprising due to the shock and multiple traumas the defendant experienced. The serum LDH levels were significantly elevated. The laboratory determined no lactate levels. The laboratory used

Abbot TDx methodology for alcohol determination in serum. This method utilizes ADH enzyme. The laboratory reported serum alcohol levels of 162 mg/dL or 0.162%.

Ricardo knew that he and his friends could not legally drink as they were below the legal age to drink. They obtained beer and went to a river to swim for a few hours. Ricardo admitted drinking beer between 2:00 p.m. and 2:30 p.m. They then left the river and were going back home when the accident happened.

14.1.4 False-Positive Blood Alcohol Levels

Because of his injuries and shock, Ricardo's blood lactate levels were expected to increase several-fold. Infusion of 3 L of Lactated Ringer's solution would further increase blood lactate considerably. Since there is no lactate utilization due to injuries, the overall blood lactate levels were expected to be extremely high at the time the blood was drawn for alcohol analysis (6,7). The laboratory analysis revealed a several-fold increase in liver enzymes including LDH.

In a normal healthy man weighing 200 pounds, one alcoholic drink is expected to give a BAC of 0.02%. Alcohol from blood is expected to dissipate at the rate of 0.02% in 1 hour (6,9). Ricardo weighed 115 pounds and admitted drinking two beers between 2:00 p.m. and 2:30 p.m. Consequently, his blood alcohol levels could go up to 0.07%. The accident occurred at approximately 7:45 p.m. There was a time lapse of approximately 5 hours from the time he drank the second beer to the time his blood was drawn. In those 5 hours, he would have eliminated any alcohol left in circulation completely. He had no alcohol in his body and was sober at the time of the accident. His serum was analyzed by the laboratory on the blood sample that was drawn at 9:46 p.m. The serum alcohol levels at this time were expected to be 0%.

The GC method of alcohol determination is the gold standard but is expensive to maintain. It has no known interferences. Several enzymatic methods by several manufacturers based on the reaction of alcohol dehydrogenase on alcohol and the conversion of NAD to NADH and extrapolating the concentration of NADH so generated to alcohol are available in the market. Several hospital laboratories use them, as they are cheaper and quicker. They are accurate in the majority of cases. But they give false-positive blood alcohol levels under certain conditions. These methods measure NADH and correlate these levels to BAC. This stoichiometric relationship is fine as long as NADH is not generated by any other enzymatic reaction. Elevated lactate and LDH in blood also generate NADH, giving false-positive blood ethanol levels (3). Several manufacturers with FDA-approved reagent kits for procedures of alcohol determination by ADH acknowledge the findings and warn about the false-positive blood alcohol levels in cases of trauma and high blood lactate and LDH levels (8).

14.1.5   Conclusions

Based on the available evidence, it can be concluded with a reasonable degree of scientific certainty that:

1. Ricardo's blood alcohol levels were falsely elevated.
2. Extremely high blood lactate and LDH levels and the use of an inappropriate enzymatic method utilizing ADH by Abbot TDx to measure serum alcohol resulted in false-positive alcohol levels.
3. Based on the evidence of the number of beers Ricardo drank, the period in which he drank, and the time of the accident, it can be concluded that he was sober at the time of the accident.
4. Alcohol had no role in the unfortunate accident resulting in the death of the doctor.

14.2   Presumptive DUI and an Injured Motorcyclist

14.2.1   Legal Aspects: Presumptive DUI and Injuries to a Motorcyclist

This case is about an accident involving a motorcycle driven by Mr. Skip Edwards who, while trying to avoid a collision with a car coming from the opposite direction on Circus road, went onto the shoulder of the road. He lost control, went into a ditch, received lacerations, and was bleeding profusely. At the Rexport Hospital emergency room, his serum alcohol was found to be 0.13%. He contends that he drank only three to four beers and there must be a mistake in his serum alcohol measurement by the hospital laboratory.

14.2.2   Medical Aspects: Falsely Elevated Alcohol Measurements by Enzymatic Methods

The enzymatic methods use the ADH and NAD to measure serum alcohol. However, elevation of serum lactate and LDH are known to occur in patients with trauma and injuries, which interferes with enzymatic methods giving rise to falsely elevated serum alcohol levels.

14.2.3   Factual Background

Skip Edwards is a Caucasian male, 42 years of age, 5 feet 11 inches tall. He weighed 190 pounds on the day of the accident. It appears that the accident happened on a clear, sunny day at 5:30 p.m. The accident took place at a bend on Circus road. Skip and his friends were at Mr. X's bar between 4:00 p.m. and 5:00 p.m. Mr. Edwards admits drinking three to four 12-oz. beers while eating a chicken dinner. He and his friends proceeded on Circus road on motorcycles with the intention of going to Mrs. Edwards's workplace. Mr. Edwards's motorcycle was the middle of the three motorcycles. Ben was riding the first motorcycle, the second motorcycle behind was that of Mr. Edwards, and the motorcycle behind him was that of Jerry. The motorcycles were going north on Circus road. The motorcycle in front was approximately 10 feet in front of Mr. Edwards's motorcycle. A car driven by Mr. Josh Combs coming in the opposite lane missed the motorcycle in front and came straight at Mr. Edwards. He had very little time to act and in order to avoid the collision, he quickly drove the motorcycle to the right side of the road to avoid impact with the car. He went off the shoulder and landed on rocks in a ditch. He was bleeding profusely and sustained multiple traumas, lacerations on the tongue and face, and a fracture in the right orbital area. The accident happened at 5:30 p.m. Since Mr. Edwards was bleeding profusely, Ben drove him on his motorcycle to his wife's place of employment and from there to Mrs. Edwards's place of work. His wife took him to Rexport Hospital emergency room. He was in the hospital for two days. His urinary drug screens were negative. His blood was drawn at the hospital at 7:45 p.m. and the alcohol levels in the serum were determined by Beckman enzymatic procedure. The serum alcohol levels were found to be 0.139%. Divide by 1.18 to get a blood alcohol level of 0.12%.

14.2.4   Cars and Motorcycle Accidents

It is generally the experience of forensic pathologists and medical examiners that operators of automobiles often do not see operators of motorcycles, either because of their low profile or because they are not attuned to looking for motorcycles. Automobiles will turn in front of a motorcycle and the motorcycle will crash into the car. Most experienced operators of motorcycles assume that individuals driving cars do not see them. Motorcycles involved in accidents always eject their operator. Generally, the motorcyclist sustains either head or neck injuries. The injuries occur from being thrown from the vehicle and hitting the ground or another object (**6**).

With the previous evidence from forensic pathology literature, it is essential to analyze the accident carefully. The three motorcycles were going on the road one after the other. The car came in suddenly at the bend and missed the first motorcycle, which was only 10 feet away from the second motorcycle driven by Mr. Edwards. This suggests that Mr. Edwards saw the car coming at him and had a few seconds to act. He was alert and quickly went to the right side, away from the car and avoided hitting it. This suggests that his mental faculties, CNS functions, and motor skills were under his control and were not consistent with a person whose blood alcohol levels

were 0.12%. Therefore, his blood alcohol levels, in all likelihood, were much
below the legal limit (6,7).

14.2.5 Blood Alcohol Levels

As stated earlier, BAC depends on several factors (6,7). In a normal healthy
individual weighing 200 pounds, one alcoholic drink is expected to result
in a blood alcohol level of 0.02%. Alcohol dissipates from blood at the rate
of 0.02% per hour (6,7). Mr. Edwards weighed 190 pounds on the day of
his accident. One 12-oz. beer was expected to give a blood alcohol level of
0.021%. He was at the bar from 4:00 p.m. to 5:00 p.m. He admits drinking 3
to 4 beers along with his chicken dinner within this one hour. The four beers
were expected to give a blood alcohol level of 0.084% at 6:00 p.m., the time at
which he was expected to reach peak blood alcohol levels. There was a time
lapse of 30 minutes from his last drink at 5:00 p.m. to the time of accident
at 5:30 p.m. In these 30 minutes, he was expected to dissipate 0.01% of alcohol from blood. This would result in 0.032% blood alcohol at the time of his
motorcycle accident. At the time of his blood draw at 7:45 p.m., a time lapse
of 2 hours and 15 minutes, he would have dissipated an additional 0.04% of
blood alcohol. This was expected to give a residual blood alcohol of 0% at
the time of his blood draw. Yet, the laboratory reports 0.139% of alcohol in
serum, which works to be 0.12% of whole blood (6). To these one has to add
0.06%, the amount that was expected to be dissipated from his blood starting
from 5:00 p.m., the time he left the bar, resulting in a blood alcohol level of
0.18%. To get these blood alcohol levels, Mr. Edwards was expected to consume between 9 to 10 beers in a matter of 1 hour while eating his dinner. This
was unlikely. He was alert and was quick to avoid the impact of his motorcycle with the car. Therefore, the four beers he reports appear to be accurate.
His behavior at the time of accident was more consistent with blood alcohol
levels of 0.04% rather than the toxic levels of 0.12%. There is an inconsistency
between the blood alcohol levels determined by the laboratory and the number of beers Mr. Edwards reports that he consumed. Mr. Edwards is reporting that he consumed four beers and the blood alcohol levels determined by
the laboratory might be falsely elevated. GC determination of blood alcohol
is the gold standard. That is why forensic blood alcohol determinations are
done by GC. Rexport Hospital laboratory is not a forensic toxicology laboratory and does not use a GC in alcohol determination. They used the Beckman
enzymatic method, which gives accurate blood alcohol levels in a majority of
cases and is enough for patient management. However, elevated circulating
lactate and LDH generated in patients with trauma are known to give false-
positive blood alcohol levels (3). Several reagent manufacturers of enzymatic
alcohol determinations now warn of this possibility in their package inserts.

14.2.6   Conclusions

It can be concluded with a reasonable degree of scientific certainty that:

1. Mr. Edwards's blood alcohol levels determined by Rexport Hospital laboratory were falsely elevated by the enzymatic method.
2. Due to Mr. Edwards' multiple traumas, lactate and LDH were released in his blood, which interfered with the enzymatic method used for serum alcohol determinations. This resulted in falsely elevated serum alcohol levels.
3. Consequently, his blood alcohol levels at the time of the accident were much below the legal limit.
4. His blood alcohol levels were such that they were not expected to cause any impairment in his judgment, motor skills, reflexes, or reaction times, and he was fit to drive.
5. This was also corroborated by the fact that with very few seconds available to him, he reacted instantaneously and immediately and avoided a collision with oncoming automobile.
6. Because of his alertness, he avoided a more serious accident to himself and to the occupants of the car.

14.3   DUI, Fatal Accident, Homicide

14.3.1   Legal Aspects: DUI and Vehicular Homicide

This case is about Mr. Rod Davilio, who lost control of his car, skidded off the highway, and ended up in a ditch hitting a tree 10-in. in diameter. Three of the occupants were ejected and were thrown out, as they were not wearing seat belts. There were serious injuries and the death of Oreana Lanan, Rod's girlfriend. The police arrested Rod Davilio for vehicular homicide and DUI. Rod contests the blood alcohol result obtained from the hospital laboratory.

14.3.2   Medical Aspects: False-Positive Blood Alcohol Levels

Serum alcohol analysis at the hospital laboratory by automatic enzymatic instrumental analysis involving ADH enzyme can give falsely elevated serum alcohol levels particularly if the patient was injured. In these patients, serum lactate dehydrogenase and lactate levels are known to be elevated. These interfere in the instrumental analysis and give false-positive serum alcohol levels. Under these circumstances, it is advisable to do serum alcohol analysis by a GC.

14.3.3 Factual Background

This motor vehicle accident involving serious injuries and a fatality happened on Saturday, March 19, 1995. According to Renagal State Police, the accident happened at 8:00 p.m.

Rod Davilio is a Caucasian male, 23 years of age, and weighing 133 pounds on the day of the accident. He was driving a 1993 Ford Mustang with his girlfriend, Oreana Lanan, 16 years of age, sitting in the front passenger seat. Joshua Lanan, 11 years of age, and Keith Clarke, 22 years of age, were in the backseat. It seems none of them was wearing seat belts. They pulled out of Quick Go store and were going to see Rod's brother. Rod was driving south on Highway 47. After a few miles, he lost control of the car, skidded off the highway, and ended up in a ditch hitting a 10-in. thick tree. Three of the passengers were ejected. Oreana was thrown in the middle of the trees and died. Joshua was seriously injured and was taken to a hospital. Keith was not seriously injured. Rod was injured and was taken to Peace on Earth Hospital. The police arrived at the accident scene at 8:47 p.m. After interviewing people at the scene, the police arrived at the hospital. Rod had lacerations and the emergency care unit treated him for these injuries. His blood was drawn by a nurse at 9:50 p.m. and the analysis of serum alcohol was done by Abbot TDX®, which gave a result of 0.13%. To convert serum alcohol levels to blood alcohol levels, 0.13% is divided by 1.1, which gave a BAC of 0.11%. He had no drugs in his system. The police arrived at the hospital and interviewed Rod at approximately 11:30 p.m. Rod had a moderate odor of alcohol on his breath, slurred speech, and unsure balance. The police arrested Rod at 12:00 a.m. for vehicular homicide and DUI, and requested Rod's blood sample, which the nurse drew for police at 12:10 a.m. The blood alcohol analyzed by the state police crime laboratory gave a reading of 0.06%. The method by which this analysis was done is not known.

14.3.4 Blood Alcohol Concentration

As stated previously, BAC depends on several factors (6,7). Rod weighed 133 pounds; one alcoholic drink is expected to give a BAC of 0.03%. At the same time, alcohol from the blood is expected to dissipate at a rate of 0.02% per hour. Rod contends that he drank only two beers at noontime at home. These two beers were expected to give a BAC of 0.06%. However, he is expected to dissipate at the rate of 0.02% per hour. Since the accident happened at 8:00 p.m., there was a time lapse of 8 hours. Therefore, the BAC due to these two beers should be 0% at 8:00 p.m. However, after the accident, the hospital drew his blood at 9:50 p.m., which showed a BAC of 0.11% (conversion of serum alcohol levels of 0.13% to BAC), and the blood drawn at the hospital for police at 12:10 a.m. gave a BAC of 0.06%. Therefore, Rod must have consumed alcoholic beverages later and possibly at a time closer to the accident.

14.3.5 Alcohol Intoxication

There is commonsense and scientific presumption that conviction should only occur if the BAC at the time of the accident is at or above the legal limit, which in turn reflects the alcohol reaching the brain, which in turn indicates the degree of acute alcohol-induced impairment of driving ability. The fact that BAC at 9:50 p.m. in the blood sample drawn at the hospital was 0.11% and in a sample drawn for police at 12:10 a.m. was 0.06% is not proof enough that Rod's BAC at the time of the accident impaired his driving ability.

BAC at 9:50 p.m. and at 12:10 a.m. contradicts his contention that he did not drink beer after he drank two beers at noontime at his home. Therefore, Rod did drink alcohol before the accident. Based on the deposition statement of several witnesses, it is possible to answer the following questions.

1. What was the possible time at which Rod consumed his last drink?
2. What was Rod's BAC at the time of the accident and its possible role in the impairment of his driving abilities?

14.3.5.1 *What Was the Possible Time at Which Rod Consumed His Last Drink?*

Deposition testimony of Rod was evasive and he never admitted drinking more beer other than the two beers he says he had around noon at his house. Therefore, it is not possible to get from him the time at which he had his last drink. He only admitted going to the Quick Go store and talking to others in the parking lot. He does not remember how long he was at the store. He remembers that Oreana and Joshua came to the store later. According to the deposition testimony of Joshua, Rod did not drink the night before. He was not drinking the whole day. According to Joshua, Rod did not appear intoxicated. Joshua further states that there was a big pothole in the road and Rod hit the pothole, lost control, and went into a ditch. According to the deposition testimony of Keith, who is Rod's cousin, Quick Go store does not care if you buy beer and drink it in your car in the parking lot if no one sees you drink. He saw Rod talking to people at the Quick Go store. According to deposition testimony of Toby Grahm, Rod was at Quick Go store. He saw the storeowner lock up the store at 7:30 p.m. He did see Rod drink beer. According to deposition testimony of Steven Blank, he saw Rod at the Quick Go store in and out of the store three times. When Rod pulled up into the parking lot, he was alone. According to Blank, he saw Rod buy a six-pack of beer. Based on this evidence, it is safe to assume that Rod did drink his last beer at 7:30 p.m., the time when Oreana and Joshua arrived at the store.

14.3.5. 2 *What Was Rod's BAC at the Time of the Accident and Its Possible Role in the Impairment of His Driving Abilities?*

From the deposition testimony of several people, it can be clearly established that Rod bought beer at Quick Go store. He probably did drink beer not seen by others, including Joshua who came to the Quick Go store when it was closing. Based on these testimonies, it can be assumed that Rod's last beer was at approximately 7:30 p.m. The accident happened very close to the Quick Go store on Highway 47. Therefore, the assumption that his last beer was at approximately 7:30 p.m. is a reasonable estimate. Based on this assumption and on the BAC at two different times, it can be concluded that Rod was still absorbing alcohol from his stomach up until the time of his first blood draw at the hospital. Evidence from the literature shows that some individuals are in the absorption phase for 2 hours or more after alcohol consumption. Based on this evidence, his BAC at various times can be calculated as follows:

Time (h)	BAC (%)	Comments
7:30 p.m.	0	Last drink at parking lot
8:00 p.m.	0.02	Accident
8:30 p.m.	0.04	
9:00 p.m.	0.06	
9:30 p.m.	0.08	
10:00 p.m.	0.10	Hospital blood draw
10:30 p.m.	0.09	
11:00 p.m.	0.08	
11:30 p.m.	0.07	
12:10 a.m.	0.06	Blood draw for police

Based on these calculations, it can be concluded with a reasonable degree of scientific certainty that Rod's BAC at the time of accident was 0 to 0.02%. It is apparent that alcohol did not play any role in the motor vehicle accident. As stated earlier, the estimated blood alcohol levels were such that they could not cause impairment of Rod's driving abilities at the time of the accident. Deposition testimony of Rod shows that the road has no shoulder where he lost control of his car. According to the deposition testimony of Joshua, there was a big pothole in the road and it is presumed that Rod hit the hole and lost control of his car. According to Mr. Blank, the road was in bad shape where the accident took place.

14.3.6 Conclusions

Based on the available facts from the medical and scientific literature, it can be concluded with a reasonable degree of scientific and medical certainty that:

1. Rod's blood alcohol levels at the time of accident were between 0 and 0.02%.
2. These blood alcohol levels cannot cause alcohol intoxication leading to impairment.
3. Alcohol had no role in this unfortunate motor vehicle accident resulting in the death of Oreana and serious injuries to Joshua.

14.4 Presumptive DUI: Car and Oil Tanker Truck Collision

14.4.1 Legal Aspects: False-Positive Blood Alcohol Levels

This case is about Veronica Bennet, who was driving her car and had a head-on collision with an oil tanker truck coming in the opposite lane. An ambulance took her to the hospital emergency room. She had multiple traumas and injuries. Based on the hospital laboratory analysis, she was arrested for presumptive DUI. She contends that her blood alcohol levels should be below the legal limit because she consumed only two beers.

14.4.2 Medical Aspects: Blood Alcohol Determinations by Enzymatic Methods

Blood alcohol measurements by automated analytical instruments involving the enzyme ADH and NAD are known to give false-positive blood alcohol levels in the presence of high serum lactate and LDH levels. In the case of Veronica, with multiple traumas and injuries, circulating lactate and LDH are expected to be elevated and give false-positive blood alcohol levels.

14.4.3 Factual Background

Veronica Bennet is a 20-year-old Caucasian female, weighing 140 pounds on the day of the collision. The accident happened at 4:20 p.m. on State Road XP 48. Veronica was the driver of the car and her friend Susan Whitesides was her passenger. The truck was driven by Skip Straightarrow, who is an experienced driver and has been driving an 18-wheeler oil truck for many years. It was drizzling and the road was wet with low visibility. Mr. Straightarrow did not sustain any injuries but the driver and the passenger of a KIA black sedan sustained multiple injuries and traumas. The driver, Veronica, suffered a concussion and became unconscious. The driver and the passenger were both pulled out of the wreck and transported to the Dellmonte Medical Center by an ambulance. During transport, the paramedic in the ambulance infused 1000 mL of Lactated Ringer's solution with an 18-gauge needle at a rate of 500 mL per hour. Upon arrival, Veronica was crying and confused, but very quickly became oriented after a brief discussion. Her right jaw was swollen, and there were lacerations on her face. It became apparent that she had multiple fractures. The attending physician, Dr. Jagan Singh, thought that her behavior immediately upon arrival at the hospital could be due to intoxication or due to closed head injury. Therefore, a blood alcohol test was ordered. Blood was drawn at 5:12 p.m. and alcohol levels in serum were determined by Kodak Ectachem 700 by ADH method at 5:50 p.m. The serum alcohol levels were found to be 241 mg/100 mL (dL) or 0.241%. This works out to be 219 mg/dL or 0.219% in whole blood. The factor to convert serum alcohol to blood alcohol was taken as 1.1 (**1**). Her blood alcohol level was twice the legal limit in the state of Xenovia.

After the accident, the police officer interviewed both Veronica and her friend Susan in the emergency room and noted that the driver of the car, Veronica, had no alcoholic smell on her breath whereas the passenger, Susan, had alcoholic breath. Because of the serious trauma and injuries, Veronica was transferred to a surgical unit.

14.4.4 Blood Alcohol Levels

BAC depends on several factors as stated earlier. In general, blood alcohol levels increase by 0.02% for one drink in a normal healthy man weighing 200 pounds. Females achieve slightly higher alcohol levels than males. It is expected that approximately 0.02% of alcohol is eliminated from the blood in one hour (**6,7**).

Veronica went to Goodtimes bar with her friend Susan at 12:45 p.m. Veronica had her first drink at 1:00 p.m. She probably had her second drink an hour later. She admitted that she had two drinks and did not have any drinks the previous day. Therefore, Veronica's blood alcohol levels should be consistent with these two drinks. Veronica weighed 140 pounds at the time of the accident. One drink would result in a blood alcohol level of 0.03%; two drinks would result in a blood alcohol level of 0.06%. She was expected to eliminate 0.02% of alcohol per hour from her blood. The accident happened at 4:20 p.m., approximately three hours after her first drink. Her blood was drawn at 5:12 p.m., one hour after the accident. Her residual alcohol level at the time of accident should be 0% and at the time of her blood draw, it should be 0%. The blood alcohol levels reported by the laboratory were 241 mg/dL or 0.241%. These alcohol levels were unrealistic numbers and there might be a serious analytical error by the method used for blood alcohol determination by the laboratory. For the sake of argument, if this value is taken as a true result, then a value of 0.08% that would be eliminated in 4 hours needs to be added to 0.241%. This works out to be 321 mg/dL or 0.321%. To get to these blood alcohol levels, Veronica would have had to consume at least 11 drinks in a matter of three hours at the bar. This is highly unlikely. Therefore, the blood alcohol levels determined by Dellmonte Medical Center were flawed.

The enzymatic method gives false-positive results (3). It was shown that elevated lactate and LDH generated in the body could also convert NAD to NADH without the presence of alcohol. It is known that lactate and LDH levels increase in injury and trauma and in various other situations. In addition, lactate is not cleared rapidly during trauma and injury (8). Kodak Company recognized these findings and clearly stated in their procedure manual that elevated lactate and LDH give false-positive blood alcohol levels and that the levels obtained in postmortem and anti-mortem blood specimens should be confirmed by GC (8).

Veronica was involved in a serous automobile accident, which resulted in her injuries, trauma, and multiple fractures. Her condition was serious enough to warrant her transfer to Dellmonte Medical Center, a well-known trauma center. The injuries she sustained would definitely result in very high circulating lactate and LDH. Moreover, she was infused with 1000 mL of Lactated Ringer's solution resulting in further elevation of lactate in her blood. Because of this high lactate and LDH, the Kodak Ektachem 700 machine gave a false-positive blood alcohol level even though she did not have any alcohol in her blood at the time of the accident.

14.4.5 Conclusions

Based on the facts, it can be concluded more probably than not that:

1. Veronica had no alcohol in her blood at the time of the accident and at the time of her blood draw.
2. The use of a method that was shown to give false-positive blood alcohol levels due to elevated lactate and LDH gave falsely elevated blood alcohol levels.
3. Thus, alcohol had no role in this unfortunate accident.

14.5 Presumptive DUI, Truck and Motorcycle Collision

14.5.1 Legal Aspects: Death of a Motorcyclist

This case is about a fatal accident involving a van and a motorcycle at 12:34 p.m. on a clear day on May 22, 2001. Lawrence Estes was driving a Honda motorcycle when a truck pulled away from the curb and came in front of him. The motorcycle crashed into the truck, which resulted in multiple traumas and the death of Lawrence. His wife, Mary, brought a civil suit against the driver of the truck, Keith Kelly for wrongful death of her husband. The defendant and his insurance company allege that Lawrence was drunk and was unfit to drive a motorcycle.

14.5.2   Medical Aspects: Falsely Elevated Pleural Cavity Alcohol Due to Contamination

The blood from the pleural cavity of the deceased gave an alcohol level of 0.12% or 120 mg/dL. Gastric fluid gave an alcohol level of 1090 mg/dL. There was no alcohol in the urine and the vitreous fluid clearly indicated contamination of the pleural cavity blood by the unabsorbed alcohol from the stomach.

14.5.3   Factual Background

The details of this accident reveal that Keith Kelly, who did not sustain any injuries, drove a 1996 Ford truck that sustained damage to the passenger side. The motorcyclist was Lawrence Estes, 33 years of age, Caucasian male, 6 feet tall and weighing 218 pounds. He was a software engineer for a university medical center. He stopped for lunch for approximately 30 minutes. His co-workers were with him for lunch. This was confirmed by the server. The server also confirmed that the decedent consumed only one beer. After lunch, Lawrence was going westbound on Atwood Street where his office was located. The truck suddenly pulled away from the curb and made a right-hand turn in front of Lawrence. The motorcycle struck the truck on the right side. Lawrence was thrown off the motorcycle and landed under the truck. This accident happened just 10 minutes after Lawrence left the lunch place. The paramedics pulled Lawrence out from beneath the truck and found him alive but unresponsive with low blood pressure. He was transported to the William Penn Hospital emergency room. He was found to be unresponsive even to pain stimuli with poor respiratory status. He was in the emergency room for 20 minutes and was then taken to the operating room. Observations in the operating room reveal that Lawrence sustained injuries to the head, chest, and spine, with multiple rib fractures. A large amount of blood was found in the left hemothorax and the stomach was clearly visible in the left chest, indicating massive disruption of the left hemi-diaphragm. Large bone fragments were found up and down the vertebral column and large amounts of blood flowed freely from this. Despite the doctor's best efforts, the patient expired. He was pronounced dead at 2:05 p.m.

14.5.4 Autopsy Report

The autopsy report needs a special comment with regard to blood alcohol (1). This autopsy was performed on May 23, 2001 at 8:20 p.m., approximately 30 hours after death. Dr. Ruben Rabin, Deputy Medical Examiner, Duchess County, Virginia, performed the autopsy. To understand the results of the autopsy, reference must be made to the hospital records. There were contusions on the lung, bilateral hemothorax, ruptured thoracic aorta, heart laceration, and brain contusion. The abdomen was protuberant. The notes written by Dr. Greg A. Martinez indicate that the stomach was clearly visible in the left chest indicating a massive disruption of the hemi-diaphragm. Moreover, large fracture fragments were found up and down the vertebral column and large amounts of blood flowed freely from this. The autopsy showed abrasions of the nose, left hip, left knee, and both ankles, and fractures of the right wrist and multiple ribs. There were 1500 ml of blood in each pleural cavity. It is significant to note that there was 700 ml of unidentified early digested food in the stomach and the urinary bladder contained 40 ml of urine. A sample of blood from the thoracic cavity, urine, vitreous fluid, and gastric fluid were sent for analysis to the toxicology laboratory. The blood from the pleural cavity gave a blood alcohol level of 0.12% or 120 mg/dL. The gastric fluid gave an alcohol level of 1090 mg/dL. There was no alcohol in the urine or the vitreous fluid. The absence of alcohol in urine and vitreous fluid clearly indicates contamination of the pleural cavity blood by the unabsorbed alcohol from the stomach (6,9).

14.5.5 Contamination of Blood from the Pleural Cavity

During severe traumatic injury when unabsorbed alcohol is present in the stomach, contamination of the blood drawn by transthoracic puncture or the blood drawn from the pleural cavity results in artificially elevated BAC. It is recommended that in cases of traumatic injury, blood from the intact heart chamber as well as blood samples from additional sites and additional body fluid be taken and analyzed for alcohol. This is to ensure that the BAC used for forensic interpretation is accurate. If alcohol from the GI tract permeates the thoracic cavity due to trauma, the samples from the chest cavity are contaminated. It is important that the BAC is representative of the circulating alcohol. A positive blood ethanol from the sample obtained from the chest cavity and the absence of alcohol in the vitreous fluid and urine suggest contamination of pleural cavity blood from unabsorbed ethanol from the stomach (6,9).

14.5.6   Blood Alcohol Concentration

As stated previously, BAC depends on several factors. A 200-pound man is expected to reach a BAC of 0.02% with one alcoholic drink (**6,7**). The decedent spent approximately 30 minutes eating lunch and had only one beer. He came out and drove his motorcycle on Atwood Street. Only 10 minutes after he left the lunch place, the truck pulled in front of him resulting in his fatal accident. Thus, the time between the decedent's drink, the fatal accident, and his death was a matter of 30 minutes. It would be impossible to attain a BAC of 0.12% after one beer (**6**). No alcohol was found in the urine, which means he was not drinking prior to arriving at the lunch place. There was no alcohol in the vitreous fluid, which means that alcohol was not absorbed into the bloodstream and diffused into the vitreous fluid. Therefore, the blood drawn from the chest cavity was contaminated from the alcohol in the stomach (**3**). The alcohol content in the stomach and the alcohol content in 3000 ml of chest blood actually add up to the alcohol in one beer. The decedent weighed 218 pounds and one beer would have given a BAC of 0.018% (**2**). To get a BAC of 0.12% as reported, the decedent had to consume at least 6 to 7 beers within 30 minutes at the lunch place.

14.5.7   Cause of the Accident

Generally, during accidents, motorcyclists sustain severe trauma including head and neck injuries. The injuries occur because of being thrown away from the vehicle and hitting the ground or another object (**6**). In this accident, the truck pulled from the curb and came suddenly in front of the motorcycle. In spite of his best efforts to stop his motorcycle, Lawrence crashed into the truck and sustained fatal injuries.

14.5.8   Conclusions

Based on the available evidence, the following conclusions can be drawn with a reasonable degree of scientific and medical certainty that:

1. Lawrence Estes was not intoxicated with alcohol and alcohol did not play any role in this fatal accident.
2. The blood obtained by the forensic pathologist from the pleural cavity was contaminated with the unabsorbed alcohol from the stomach.
3. The accident was caused by the negligence of the truck driver who pulled his truck from the curb in front of the motorcycle.
4. The driver of the truck bears responsibility for the untimely and unnecessary death of Lawrence Estes.

14.6   DUI, Alcohol, and Tylenol

14.6.1   Legal Aspects: False-Positive Blood Alcohol

This case is about Stanley Hathook, who was involved in traffic accident where his Jeep lost control and hit a mailbox and a pole. The police arrested him for presumptive DUI. However, Stanley contends that he drank only two beers and his blood alcohol level must be below the legal limit.

14.6.2   Medical Aspects: Tylenol and False-Positive Blood Alcohol

The liver metabolizes both Tylenol and alcohol. Drinking alcohol when taking Tylenol reduces the metabolism of alcohol and consequently elevates blood alcohol levels. Taking Tylenol and drinking alcohol may lead to liver failure.

14.6.3   Factual Background

Mr. Stanley Hathook is a 25-year-old Caucasian male, weighing 200 pounds on April 30, 2000, the day of his accident and his arrest by the police for possible DUI. The defendant was driving his Jeep on State Road 63, lost control of the vehicle, and struck a mailbox and a pole at approximately 12:15 p.m. The defendant was thrown out onto the paved road and sustained a blow to the left side of his head. He also sustained cuts and bruises on his knee and on other places on his body. The defendant used the telephone of the property owner at the accident site and notified his girlfriend. His girlfriend drove him home. The defendant admits that he drank one beer at home at approximately 11:45 a.m. prior to the accident. It is relevant to note that the defendant is a regular beer drinker and says that he drinks 10 to 12 beers per week. Two days prior to his accident, the defendant injured his right middle finger with a sledgehammer at work and saw his doctor at 3:00 p.m. He has been taking Tylenol every four hours and says that he probably took eight tablets that day. He telephoned the police about the accident from his home. The police arrived at his home and the defendant says that the police saw him drinking at his home. The defendant was transferred to the hospital and was interviewed by police at 2:40 p.m. On suspicion of possible DUI, the police requested that two tubes of blood be drawn from the defendant. Tubes of blood were drawn at 2:50 p.m. by the hospital technologist and were sent to the State Police Erie Regional Laboratory where the blood was analyzed for alcohol by headspace GC. The blood alcohol level was found to be 0.258%.

14.6.4   Blood Alcohol Levels

BAC depends on several factors as elucidated earlier (**6,8**). The defendant weighed 200 pounds and consumed one 16-oz. beer at home at 11:45 a.m. prior to the accident. A 16-oz. beer is expected to result in a blood alcohol level of 0.026% at the time of the accident. This level would not be expected to result in intoxication in a regular beer drinker. Yet, he lost control of his Jeep and was involved in an accident. One of the possible reasons might be the synergistic toxicity of eight tablets of acetaminophen and alcohol. Subsequent to his accident, he went home and drank six beers. Six beers are expected to give a blood alcohol level of 0.156%, from which 0.06% need to be subtracted to take the dissipation of alcohol in three hours at a rate of 0.02% per hour into consideration. The blood draw was at 2:50 p.m. Therefore, his final blood alcohol level was expected to be 0.096%. However, the laboratory reported a blood alcohol level of 0.258%. This discrepancy needs to be reconciled. The police laboratory used a GC. The value as reported by the laboratory appears to be accurate and there are no grounds to challenge this result. This discrepancy can be explained by the combined and synergistic toxicity of Tylenol and alcohol.

14.6.5   Tylenol, Alcohol, and Liver Failure

It is indeed fortunate that the defendant did not die. He lost control of the Jeep he was driving, was thrown out onto the paved road, and escaped with a few bumps and bruises. He took eight tablets of Tylenol and drank six beers, a dangerous toxic combination. He was nauseated and vomiting, suggesting that he developed acute liver toxicity and fortunately recovered without liver failure. The defendant drinks beer regularly and can be considered a chronic alcohol user. Alcoholics are predisposed to acetaminophen toxicity (**10-12**).

Alcohol as well as fasting enhances hepatic toxicity of even small doses of acetaminophen (**5**). Severe acetaminophen toxicity in chronic alcoholics by intake of alcohol has been reported. Moreover, acetaminophen hepatotoxicity appears to be increased in humans and in experimental animals by prior alcohol abuse (**11**). For these reasons, alcoholics should be cautioned about the simultaneous use of acetaminophen. Acetaminophen toxic symptoms include neuralgic signs and coma, hematological abnormalities, pancreatitis, vomiting, and liver failure. Nausea and vomiting may occur 12 to 14 hours later. Thus, ethanol enhances acetaminophen toxicity even with small doses and it appears that acetaminophen inhibits ADH, an enzyme involved in the metabolism of alcohol, and decreases its clearance from blood. Consequently, acetaminophen elevates blood alcohol levels (**10-12**).

Thus, the defendant, a regular alcohol user, took nearly 8 to 10 tablets of Tylenol and drank one beer prior to the accident. This combination is enough to enhance the toxicity of Tylenol and probably resulted in neurologic problems leading to the loss of his coordination even when the blood alcohol levels were not more than 0.026%. A level of 0.258% alcohol at blood draw as reported by the police laboratory can be explained by the fact that the Tylenol tablets he took inhibited the clearance of alcohol from blood and elevated their levels (**10–12**). If, indeed, the number of beers the defendant drank prior to the accident as well as after the accident are correctly reported, then the defendant's blood alcohol levels at the time of the accident would be below the legal limit. He was not intoxicated due to alcohol but suffered toxicity of Tylenol.

14.6.6   Conclusions

It can be concluded with a reasonable degree of scientific certainty that:

1. The defendant's blood alcohol levels were much below the legal limit at the time he was involved in the accident.
2. The defendant suffered Tylenol toxicity and was lucky to be alive without going into liver failure.

References

1. Burtis, C.A., Ashwood, E.R., and Burns, D.E. (Eds.) *Tietz Textbook of Clinical Chemistry and Molecular Biology*, 4th ed. W.B. Saunders Company, Philadelphia, PA, 2006.
2. Jortani, S.A. and Poklis, A. Emit ETS plus ethyl alcohol assay for the determination of ethyl alcohol in human serum and urine. *J. Anal. Toxicol.* **16**:368–71, 1993.
3. Nine, J.S., Moraca, M., Virji, M.A., and Rao, K.N. Serum-ethanol determination: Comparison of lactate and lactate dehydrogenase interference in three enzymatic assays. *J. Analytical Toxicol.* **19**:192–196, 1995.
4. Abramson, D., Scales, T.M., Hitchock, R., Troooskin, S.Z., Henry, S.M., and Greenspaan, J. Lactate clearance and survival following injury. *J. Trauma* **35**:584–590, 1993.
5. Didwania, A., Miller, J., Kassel, D., Jackson, E.V., and Chernow, B. Effect of lactated Ringer's solution infusion on the circulating lactate concentration: Part 3. Results of respective, randomized double-blind, placebo-controlled trial. *Crit. Care Med.* **25**:1851–1854, 1997.
6. DiMaio, V.J. and DiMaio, D. *Forensic Pathology*, 2nd ed. CRC Press, Boca Raton, FL, 2001, 516–519.
7. Williams, R.H. and Leikin, T. Medico-legal issues and specimen collection for ethanol testing. *Lab. Med.* **30**:630–637, 1999.
8. Test Methodology. Alcohol VITROS. Procedure Manual, Johnson & Johnson Clinical Diagnostics, Rochester, NY, 1996, 1–10.
9. Winek Jr., L.L., Winek, L.L., and Whaba, W.W. The role of trauma in postmortem blood alcohol determination. *Forensic Sci. Int.* **71**:1–8, 1995.

10. Seifert, C.F., Lucas, D.S., Vondracek, T.G., Kastens, D.J., McCarty, D.L., and Bui, B. Patterns of acetaminophen use in alcoholics. *Pharmacotherapy.* **13**:391–395, 1993.
11. Whitcomb, D.C. and Block, G.D. Association of acetaminophen hepatotoxicity with fasting and ethanol use. *J. Am. Med. Assoc.* **272**:1845–1850, 1994.
12. Zimmerman, H.J. and Maddrey, W.C. Acetaminophen (paracetamol) hepatotoxicity with regular intake of alcohol: analysis of instances of therapeutic misadventure. *Hepatology.* **22**:767–773, 1995.

Alcohol and Drugs $\quad$ 15

This chapter is about the synergistic effects of alcohol and drugs. These effects are highlighted with examples of several case studies. Synergism is the capacity of two or more drugs acting together so that the total effect of these drugs is greater than the sum of the two drugs acting alone and independently. These cases are about interaction of alcohol and prescription as well as over-the-counter medications. Doctors and pharmacies instruct patients not to drink alcohol when on certain medications. For example, drugs that affect or suppress the CNS should not be used simultaneously with alcohol. This simultaneous use can cause a synergistic reaction leading to fatal consequences (1-3).

15.1 DUI, Injured Cyclist

15.1.1 Legal Aspects: DUI and Injured Cyclist

This report deals with an accident involving a 14-year-old boy, Billy Bella, who was hit by a pickup truck while he was riding his bike. The accident resulted in serious injuries and fractures to the cyclist. The pickup truck was driven by David Palmer, of Palmer Constructions, Inc. The police arrested Mr. Palmer for presumptive DUI. The family of the cyclist, Billy Bella, brought a civil lawsuit against Mr. Palmer and Palmer Construction Company for monetary compensation for pain and suffering of the cyclist. Mr. Palmer admits drinking alcohol while he was on prescription medications.

15.1.2 Medical Aspects: Alcohol and Synergistic Effect of Prescription Medications

Alcohol is metabolized by the liver and the synergistic effects of prescription medications on alcohol intoxication are well known. For this reason, patients on certain prescription medications are advised not to drink alcohol.

15.1.3 Factual Background

This report deals with an accident involving a 14-year-old bicyclist and a pickup truck. The accident happened on July 24, 2005, resulting in serious injuries to the bicyclist.

Billy Bella is a Caucasian male, 14 years of age, living at home with his parents Robert and Susan. He was attending Taylor High School and completed 9th grade. He was on summer vacation. On July 24, 2005, he was riding his bicycle with his family friend Joseph, who also was riding his bicycle. Billy was wearing a helmet. At approximately 3:00 p.m., both boys were riding their bikes in the parking lot at 35 Sawmill Run Road, Wellwood, Karentakey. This parking lot connects to a bike path, which connects with a small wooden bridge. It was a clear, sunny day. David Palmer was driving a Red Dodge Ram pickup truck. The pickup truck first backed up into a parking space and then came forward. The driver's side of the bumper of the truck hit the front tire of Billy's bicycle and his left knee. Billy fell down on his back and was in intense pain. His friend Joseph saw it happen. Billy was bleeding. Joseph and David Palmer put Billy in the pickup truck and drove him home. Mr. Palmer told Billy's parents that he felt sorry for the accident. The police came to Billy's house and spoke to Billy's parents. An ambulance was called in, which took Billy to Sanjeev Hospital emergency room.

The accident resulted in serious injuries and health consequences to Billy requiring hospitalization and physical therapy. His knee was fractured and the orthopedic doctor gave him a knee immobilizer. He was confined to home for eight weeks. Because of the injuries to his back, he developed an infection, which required a visit to the emergency room and treatment at the hospital. This disabled Billy for several weeks.

David Palmer is a Caucasian male, 44 years of age, 5 feet 10 inches tall and weighing approximately 175 pounds. He is the president of Palmer Construction. He admitted to the police that he is on prescription medications, which included Wellbutrin for depression, Altace for high blood pressure, and Asacol for ulcerative colitis. He took all these medicines in the morning with breakfast. The dosages of these medications were not given. In his testimony, Mr. Palmer said that he had breakfast that day and started working at 8:30 a.m. He had a chicken salad sandwich for lunch at 12:00 p.m. He also had a snack in the afternoon. He admitted purchasing a bottle of white wine. He said that he consumed approximately 1½ glasses of white wine starting with his lunch. However, according to the testimony of Billy's parents, they said that Mr. Palmer smelled of alcohol and was drunk when he was at their house. The police assured them that they would investigate. The police also told them that Mr. Palmer admitted drinking two or three glasses of wine. The police gave Mr. Palmer field sobriety tests but no Breathalyzer test. No police intoxication report was available.

15.1.4   Alcohol, Medications, and Cognitive Functions

Alcohol and several medications alone or in combination impair cognitive functions. Ethanol, also called ethyl alcohol or alcohol, is a water-soluble compound, and readily distributes into several body compartments including the brain. BAC correlates well with the alcohol levels reaching the brain, which reflect the level of alcohol intoxication. As stated previously, BAC depends upon several factors (3-11). Patients are advised not to consume alcohol when they are on certain prescription medications. Mr. Palmer is an educated person; he has a 4-year college degree. Yet, he was irresponsible in drinking alcohol while taking Wellbutrin, Altace, and Asacol.

15.1.4.1   *Wellbutrin*

Wellbutrin is prescribed for depression. This drug is also known as bupropion. It has a half-life of 4 to 24 hours. It is protein bound in plasma and remains in circulation for a long time (7). This medication has side effects and can make a person drowsy and dizzy. Alcohol may make the side effects of this drug worse. This drug clearly interacts with alcohol and may interfere with its clearance (6-8). In fact, there is a published case report that showed the combination of bupropion and alcohol resulted in a fatality (8). People taking this drug are asked to operate motor vehicles and machinery with caution. Patients taking this medication are asked not to drink alcohol (6-8).

Altace is prescribed for high blood pressure. Side effects include drowsiness and dizziness. Patients taking this drug should avoid alcohol because it could further lower blood pressure and increase drowsiness or dizziness (7,8).

15.1.5   Alcohol Intoxication

Based on Mr. Palmer's testimony, he bought a bottle of white wine and drank 1½ glasses. According to Billy's parents, the police told them that Mr. Palmer admitted drinking 2 to 3 glasses of wine. Since he had lunch and was snacking in the afternoon, there was food in his stomach. In addition to the food in the stomach, the medication with a long half-life delays alcohol clearance. Mr. Palmer weighed 175 pounds. It is assumed that he drank two 8-oz. glasses of wine. White wine is assumed to have 15% alcohol content. Based on these assumptions, it is possible to calculate Mr. Palmer's BAC at the time of the accident.

It is scientifically accepted that a 150-pound man will have a BAC of 0.025% after drinking 1 oz. of 50% alcohol (6). Given this assumption, which is accurate under almost all circumstances, the BAC of Mr. Palmer can be calculated as follows:

$$BAC = 150 \div \text{Body weight} \times \% \text{ ethanol content} \div 50 \times \text{ounces consumed} \times 0.025$$

$$BAC \text{ of Mr. Palmer} = 150 \div 175 \times 15 \div 50 \times 16 \times 0.025 = 0.10\%$$

Based on these calculations, Mr. Palmer's BAC was 0.1% at the time of the accident, which was above the legal limit of 0.08% in the state of Karentakey. He was intoxicated with alcohol even without taking into consideration the synergistic effects of Wellbutrin and Altace. At this BAC, a person experiences impairment of sensory-motor activities, reaction times, attention, visual acuity, and judgment. The individual may still appear sober (**3**).

15.1.6   Conclusions

Based on the available evidence, it can be concluded with a reasonable degree of medical and scientific certainty that:

1. Mr. Palmer drank alcohol while on prescription medications even though he was fully aware that the combination of alcohol and his medications would seriously impair his cognitive functions.
2. Mr. Palmer was intoxicated and was unfit to drive and operate his pickup truck at the time of the accident.
3. Mr. Palmer bears full responsibility for the accident.
4. The accident caused serious trauma and injuries to Billy Bella resulting in his pain and suffering and his disability for a considerable amount of time.

15.2   Presumptive DUI, Drug Synergistic Toxicity

15.2.1   Legal Aspects: Presumptive DUI and Possession of a Controlled Substance

This case is about Mr. Aaron Asky, who was stopped by the police and was arrested for presumptive DUI and possession of controlled substances. The police officer searched and found in the pockets of the defendant five small green pills and four white rocks, which were presumed to be crack cocaine. The green pills were identified as Valium. The defendant's BAC was determined to be 0.04% and no cocaine or other drugs of abuse were reported in the serum. Diazepam and nordiazepam levels were in the therapeutic range. He was not charged with DUI but was sentenced for possession of crack cocaine.

15.2.2   Medical Aspects: Synergistic Toxicity of Alcohol and Controlled Substances

The defendant's BAC was only 0.04%, which is considered a subclinical level. He had no cocaine in the serum and his diazepam and nordiazepam levels were in the therapeutic range. This and his BAC cannot cause intoxication.

15.2.3 Factual Background

The defendant, Aaron Asky, is a Caucasian male, 6 feet tall and weighing 210 pounds on October 1, 2004, the day on which he was stopped by the police at approximately 2:30 p.m. and charged with possible DUI and possession of a controlled substance. The defendant was driving a silver Toyota Camry traveling east on Belaware Pike. He worked from 4:00 a.m. to 12:00 p.m. and stopped at his sister's place for pizza and a couple of beers before driving to his home. The police officer stopped the defendant on suspicion that he was driving his vehicle at an excessive rate of speed. According to the officer, the defendant had a mild odor of alcoholic breath. The preliminary breath test (PBT) administered by the officer gave a reading of 0.057%. It appears that the officer, frustrated with the low presumptive BAC, searched the defendant's pockets and found five small green pills. The officer also discovered four white rocks, which were presumed to be crack cocaine. Mr. Asky was subsequently taken to Blue Lagoon Hospital where his blood was drawn at 3:00 p.m. by a hospital technician.

The tubes of blood, the green pills, and the white rock substance obtained from the defendant were submitted for laboratory analysis. State Police Regional Laboratory identified the green pills as diazepam and the white chunky powder to be 0.8 g of cocaine. Mr. Asky's serum was sent to MedScan for quantitation of BAC, which was found to be 41 mg/dL or 0.04%. The serum was also used for immunochemical detection of diazepam and nordiazepam. These two compounds were further quantitated by GC-MS. The serum contained 356 ng/ml of diazepam and 182 ng/ml of nordiazepam. The laboratory could not detect opiates, barbiturates, cocaine, amphetamines, cannabinoids, PCP, or methaqualone by immunochemical assay in serum.

15.2.4 Blood Alcohol Concentration

As stated previously, BAC depends on several factors. In a normal healthy male weighing 200 pounds, one alcoholic drink is expected to give a BAC of 0.02% (3,10). In the same individual, alcohol from blood dissipates at a rate of 0.02% per hour (3). The defendant's blood was used to measure alcohol by an enzymatic procedure as well as by headspace GC. The result was a BAC of 0.04%.

Blood alcohol levels reflect the levels reaching the brain and this in turn reflects the level of alcohol intoxication. There is a commonsense and scientific presumption that conviction should only occur if the BAC, and subsequently the alcohol reaching the brain, indicates alcohol-induced impairment of driving ability. A BAC between 0.01 to 0.05% is considered sub-clinical and the majority of the population do not have any physical or mental impairment (3,9). According to the law in Pennsylvania, the levels are far below the legal limit.

15.2.4.1   Valium (Diazepam)

Diazepam is effective in the management of generalized anxiety disorders and panic disorder. This drug is also used in the treatment of skeletal muscle spasms due to inflammation or trauma. This drug can become addictive (7,8). The half-lives of serum diazepam and its metabolite nordiazepam are 21 to 37 hours and 50 to 99 hours, respectively (7). The therapeutic serum levels are 0.142 to 1 µg/ml. Based on several studies, peak plasma diazepam levels were determined to be 253 to 568 ng/ml. Peak serum levels occur in 0.5 to 2.5 hours after intake. Benzodiazepines are generally of low order toxicity. Death from overdose ingestion of benzodiazepines alone is extremely rare (7,12). According to another study, the therapeutic diazepam serum levels are 0.02 to 4.0 µg/ml and toxic levels are 5 to 20 µg/ml; greater than 30 µg/ml is considered lethal (7,8). Based on a standard pharmacology textbook, diazepam can cause CNS depression at 900 to 1000 ng/ml (12-14).

The defendant's serum was found to contain 346 ng/ml of diazepam and 182 ng/ml of nordiazepam. These levels are in the therapeutic range and much below toxic levels. Moreover, this drug can cause CNS depression, which can occur only when serum levels are at 0.9 to 1.0 µg/ml (14,15). Mr. Askey's benzodiazepine levels were much below the levels to cause CNS depression; therefore, these levels could not cause impairment of his driving abilities.

The defendant's blood alcohol concentration was 0.04%. These levels are considered sub-clinical and are expected not to cause any physical impairment of driving ability. Similarly, the serum levels of diazepam and nordiazepam are within the therapeutic levels and were much below the levels that lead to CNS depression. They were not in the toxic range.

15.2.5   Conclusions

It can be concluded with a reasonable degree of medical and scientific certainty that:

1. The defendant's blood alcohol levels were 0.04%, which is definitely sub-clinical levels and are not expected to cause any alcohol intoxication leading to impairment of driving ability.
2. The serum diazepam and nordiazepam concentrations were at low therapeutic levels and were much below the levels that cause CNS depression.
3. The defendant was not intoxicated with ethanol or with diazepam. He had no impairment whatsoever in his driving ability.

15.3   DUI, Drugs, and Leaving the Scene of an Accident

15.3.1   Legal Aspects: DUI and Drug Interaction

This case is about Ms. Kranti Kensisky, who was arrested for leaving the scene of an accident and on suspicion of presumptive DUI. Kranti contends that she was not aware of the accident and her BAC could not be as high as 0.21 as the state police laboratory analysis suggests. She said that she had only two vodkas with water. She had taken two tablets of ibuprofen and she was on naproxen. The two medications might have affected her BAC.

15.3.2   Medical Aspects: Synergistic Toxicity of Naproxen and Alcohol

Naproxen and consumption of alcoholic drinks have impaired Kranti's judgment with respect to leaving the scene of the accident. Naproxen alone can cause these behavioral abnormalities even at therapeutic doses in some individuals. The combined use of alcohol and naproxen can synergistically further enhance these effects.

15.3.3   Factual Background

Kranti Kensisky is a 50-year-old Caucasian female, weighing 114 pounds on February 23, 1999, the day of the accident and her arrest by the state police for possible DUI. The accident happened at approximately 8:55 p.m. The defendant was driving a Honda Accord 1998, on State Road XY8 toward the intersection with Queens Road. The defendant's vehicle went into the opposite lane, closely missed another vehicle, and struck the driver side of the vehicle driven by Julie Desai. Several motorists witnessed this accident. The defendant left the scene of the accident and drove to a friend's house. The police caught up with her at the friend's house. The police found her with alcoholic breath, confused, and somewhat disoriented. The defendant swayed and her walking was unsure. The defendant admitted that she drank two vodkas and water at Tipps Cove Bar. The police administered a breath alcohol test and estimated her BAC to be 0.21%. The defendant claimed that she was a responsible citizen and insisted that she was not aware of the accident. She stated that the combination of prescribed medication, naproxen, and consumption of alcoholic drinks might have impaired her judgment with regard to leaving the scene of the accident. She also took two tablets of ibuprofen on the day of the accident. She further contends that in no way could she have known about the accident. She was undergoing therapy for neuroma of her right foot.

15.3.4   Blood Alcohol Concentration

BAC depends on several factors as stated previously (**3,11**). People with end-stage liver disease accumulate very high BAC even when they drink non-alcoholic beer (**16**). Medications affecting liver function also tend to increase BAC (**3-11**). In a normal healthy male weighing 200 pounds, one alcoholic drink results in BAC of 0.02%. At the same time, 0.02% of BAC is dissipated from blood in 1 hour (**3**). Since the defendant weighed 114 pounds, one alcoholic drink should result in a BAC of 0.035%. The two drinks she admits she drank should result in a BAC of 0.07%. However, the breath alcohol test administered by the police estimated her BAC to be 0.21%. There are no grounds to challenge the accuracy of this test.

It is most likely that the elevated BAC levels were due to the naproxen she was taking. Patients are warned not to consume alcohol while taking non-steroidal medications like naproxen (**17**). A BAC of 0.21% can cause emotional instability, lack of critical judgment, impairment of memory, and comprehension (**8**). Naproxen alone can cause these behavioral abnormalities even at therapeutic doses in some individuals (**8**). The combined use of alcohol and naproxen can synergistically further enhance these effects.

15.3.4.1   *Naproxen*

The defendant started taking naproxen three days before the accident. She as well as her physician did not have time to evaluate the adverse effects of this drug. Naproxen is a non-steroidal anti-inflammatory drug that is used to alleviate pain and inflammation (**8**). This drug is nearly 100% absorbed from the GI tract. The half-life of this drug is 13 hours with a volume of distribution of 0.1L/kg. Naproxen is metabolized mainly by the liver and is excreted through the kidneys. Naproxen was shown to cause hepatotoxicity with alcohol as evidenced by elevation of liver enzymes (**18-20**). Consequently, the Food and Drug Administration has recommended that patients taking naproxen should not drink alcoholic beverages (**17**). Naproxen can also cause adverse reactions even at therapeutic doses in some individuals. These include CNS effects such as dizziness, drowsiness, and vertigo. Naproxen was also shown to cause cognitive dysfunction, such as forgetfulness, inability to concentrate, depression, disorientation, and paranoid ideation (**21,22**).

15.3.5   Conclusions

It can be concluded with a reasonable degree of scientific certainty that:

1. The defendant should not have consumed alcohol when she was on naproxen.

2. Naproxen and alcohol compete for metabolism by the liver and consequently it is not surprising that her BAC was elevated to 0.21% even though she only had two drinks.
3. Combined use of naproxen and alcohol caused synergistic toxicity and resulted in her CNS effects and cognitive dysfunction.
4. It is probable that she was not in a position to comprehend the consequences of her actions when she left the scene of the accident.
5. Naproxen-induced synergistic toxicity combined with alcohol caused these behavioral problems.

15.4 Elevated Blood Alcohol Due to Medications

15.4.1 Legal Aspects: Alcohol and Prescription Medications

This case is about Mr. Meson Geramid, who was stopped by the police on suspicion of presumptive DUI. He was given field sobriety tests, which he failed. He was arrested and his blood was sent for analysis of alcohol. Blood analysis showed that Mr. Geramid had a BAC of 0.16%. Mr. Geramid contends that he drank only two or three shots of vodka and the blood alcohol analysis is flawed.

15.4.2 Medical Aspects: Elevated Blood-Alcohol Due to Prescription Medications

The prescription medications might interact with alcohol metabolism by the liver resulting in falsely elevated blood alcohol levels.

15.4.3 Factual Background

Mr. Meson Geramid is 66 years of age. He is a Caucasian male, 5 feet 8 inches tall and weighing 193 pounds on the day of his arrest for possible DUI. Mr. Geramid has a crocodile farm and exports crocodile meat and skin. He also owns several racehorses. He was driving a 2000 Cadillac Sedan. He was staying at Full Moon Cottage. He drank two or three vodkas that evening. He started drinking at 8:00 p.m., finished his last drink at 9:30 p.m., and then left the cottage immediately. On his way home, he stopped at a restaurant and asked for directions. The people at the restaurant called 911 and alerted them about Mr. Geramid and the car he was driving. According to the police arrest report, Skyloop County 911 alerted the police to look for a dark-colored Cadillac. The police stopped Mr. Geramid and gave him field sobriety tests, which he failed. He was arrested and taken to County Medical Center. Blood was drawn at 11:13 p.m. and the blood alcohol analysis gave a result of

0.16%. Mr. Geramid told the police that he was taking prescription medications daily. He was on 250 mg of Depakote, three times a day, 20 mg capsule of Prozac, once a day, and 5 mg of Norvasc.

15.4.4   Blood Alcohol Concentration

BAC depends upon several factors as previously mentioned. In a normal healthy male weighing 200 pounds, one alcoholic drink gives a BAC of 0.02%. Alcohol in blood is dissipated at a rate of 0.02% in one hour in a normal healthy male (3,4). Patients with end-stage liver disease cannot metabolize alcohol and their blood alcohol levels become elevated even if they drink non-alcoholic beer (16). Mr. Geramid is on prescription medications and they clearly affected the metabolism of alcohol.

Prozac is an antidepressant and it is essentially metabolized by the liver with a long elimination plasma half-life. Because Prozac may impair judgment, thinking, or motor skills, patients taking this medication are advised not to drive or operate dangerous machinery. Both Prozac and alcohol depress the CNS. Therefore, patients taking this medication are advised not to drink (5).

Depakote is metabolized by the liver with a plasma half-life of 9 to 16 hours. Patients taking this medication are advised not to drive a motor vehicle. They are also advised not to drink. Both Depakote and alcohol produce CNS depression. Norvasc is a long-acting calcium channel blocker. It is also completely metabolized by the liver with a long plasma elimination half-life (8).

Mr. Geramid was advised not to drive a motor vehicle as Prozac and Depakote can depress the CNS and greatly inhibit his judgment and motor skills. He was also advised not to drink while he is on these medications as alcohol can also cause CNS depression and will inhibit his motor skills and judgment. The prescription medications and alcohol have additive and synergistic effects. They inhibited his judgment and motor skills. Even though Mr. Geramid is accustomed to drinking alcoholic beverages daily, he is not immune to the synergistic effects of prescription medications and alcohol.

Mr. Geramid claims that he drank only two or three vodkas that evening, and his BAC as determined by the hospital approximately 3.5 hours after his first drink was 0.16%. Three vodkas for Mr. Geramid weighing 193 pounds would give a maximum BAC of 0.06%. Mr. Geramid was expected to metabolize 0.02% of alcohol from blood in 1 hour. After a lapse of 3 hours, he was expected to metabolize 0.06%. Therefore, his BAC at 11:13 p.m. should have been 0%. To get 0.16% BAC, Mr. Geramid would have had to consume at least 11 shots of vodka (one shot of vodka, which is 1.5 oz., has same amount of alcohol as in a 12-oz. can of beer with 5% alcohol) between 8:00 p.m. and 9:30 p.m., the time at which he left the cottage. Either he is under-reporting the number of vodkas he consumed or he is not dissipating alcohol from his blood due to his prescription medications, Prozac and Depakote. These two medications compete with alcohol in its metabolism in liver. Therefore, even with two or three vodkas his BAC could have been artificially elevated, in which case he would show symptoms of intoxication due to the combined and synergistic actions of Prozac, Depakote, and alcohol. This is not surprising because people with end-stage liver disease can reach high BAC even if they drink non-alcoholic beer (16). Therefore, Mr. Geramid's BAC was artificially elevated. He is not supposed to drink alcohol or drive a motor vehicle when he is on Prozac and Depakote.

15.4.5   Conclusions

It can be concluded with a reasonable degree of scientific certainty that:

1. Mr. Geramid's BAC of 0.16% is artificially elevated due to his prescription medications.
2. Without these medications, his BAC for three vodkas at 11:13 p.m. should have been 0%.
3. At the time the police stopped him at 9:48 p.m., his BAC should have been 0.03%.
4. He should not have driven his car after he consumed alcohol particularly when he was taking Prozac and Depakote.

15.5   Alcohol and Prescription Medications

15.5.1   Legal Aspects: DUI

This case is about a defendant who was stopped by the police at a DUI checkpoint. His BAC of 0.083% was determined by headspace GC. Since this is just above the legal limit (0.08%), he was arrested for DUI. The defendant says that his BAC cannot be nearly as high as the test results suggest. He says that there must be a mistake in the laboratory analysis based on the number of beers he drank and the time between his last beer and his blood draw.

15.5.2   Medical Aspects: Differences between Calculated and Analytical Values of BAC

It is possible to calculate the expected BAC based on the body weight, the number of drinks consumed and their alcoholic content, and the period in which they were consumed. All methods for blood alcohol measurement are subject to 5 to 10% statistical variation. This is important when the BAC is on the borderline for the legal limit.

15.5.3 Factual Background

Daniel Gilcrist is a 36-year-old Caucasian male. He weighs 280 pounds and is 5 feet 11 inches tall. He attended a Pittsburgh Penguins and Philadelphia Flyers hockey game on September 29, 2007 and drank two 12-oz. Coors Light beers at the game. His first beer at the game was at 7:15 p.m. and he drank the second beer at 9:00 p.m. He also ate a hot dog. He says that he left the game at 10:00 p.m. and went to a tavern with a friend. He had three more 12-oz. cans of Coors Light beer. His third beer was at 11:00 p.m., the fourth beer was at 12:00 a.m., and the fifth beer was at 1:15 a.m. He left the tavern at 2:00 a.m. He was driving a Dodge Dart Sedan and was stopped by the police at a DUI checkpoint at 2:45 a.m. The police reported that Daniel failed field sobriety tests. His blood was drawn at 3:08 a.m. and was sent for blood alcohol analysis to the PAT Forensic Laboratory. The analysis performed by headspace GC gave a BAC of 0.083%.

15.5.4 Blood Alcohol Concentration

Ethanol, also called ethyl alcohol or alcohol, is a water-soluble compound that readily distributes into several body compartments including the brain. BAC reflects the alcohol reaching the brain and this in turn reflects the level of alcohol intoxication. BAC depends on the number of drinks consumed, their alcohol content, and the time frame in which they were consumed. BAC also depends upon the time lapse between the last drink and the time at which the BAC was measured. In addition, BAC depends on body weight, age, gender, health, and use of prescription or over-the-counter medications. It takes between 60 and 90 minutes for alcohol to be completely absorbed from the GI tract and reach peak levels in the blood. In some individuals, this is known to take more than two hours. Food in the stomach is known to delay absorption. Alcohol is metabolized by the liver and is dissipated from the blood at a rate of 0.02 % per hour (3,4).

15.5.5 Calculation of BAC

It is scientifically accepted that a 150-pound man will have a BAC of 0.025% after drinking 1 oz. of 100 proof (50%) alcohol. This assumption is accurate under almost all circumstances (6). The following equation is used to calculate BAC.

$$BAC = 150 \div \text{Body weight} \times \% \text{ ethanol content} \div 50 \times \text{Ounces consumed} \times 0.025$$

Daniel weighed 280 pounds on the day of the incident. He says that he drank Coors Light beer, which has an alcoholic content of 4.2%. He drank 12-oz. cans of beer. Based on this information, his calculated BAC would be as follows:

$$\text{BAC due to 1 beer} = 150 \div 280 \times 4.2 \div 50 \times 12 \times 0.025 = 0.013\%$$

$$\text{BAC due to 5 beers} = 0.065\%$$

Daniel admits drinking five beers. His first beer at the game was at 7:15 p.m., the second beer was at 9:00 p.m., and he had a hot dog at this time. He left the game at 10:00 p.m. and went to a tavern with a friend. His third beer was at 11:00 p.m., the fourth beer was at 12:00 a.m., and the fifth beer was at 1:15 a.m. He left the tavern at 2:00 a.m. His blood draw at the DUI checkpoint was at 3:08 a.m. Thus, there was a time lapse of at least two hours between his last beer and his blood draw. In these two hours, he was expected to dissipate 0.04% of alcohol from his blood. If this were subtracted from 0.065%, his resultant BAC would be 0.025%. The discrepancy between this calculated value and the BAC determined by the GC might be due to the prescription medications. Mr. Gilcrist was taking prescription medications for the past year. The medications include Lexapro, 20 mg/day, Wellbutrin, 100 mg/day, Lasix, 40 mg/day, and Cytomel, 500 µg twice a day. These prescription medications as well as alcohol are metabolized by the liver and they tend to slow down the dissipation of alcohol from blood (4,13).

15.5.6 Accuracy and Precision of Blood Alcohol Analysis by Headspace GC

Accuracy and precision are extremely important for blood alcohol determination in a clinical laboratory as well as in a forensic laboratory. Patient management in a clinical setting as well as conviction by law enforcement depends on the blood alcohol result. GC determination of blood alcohol is considered a gold standard, as the method is subjected to very few analytical inferences (12,23). Even then, the result is subject to human errors as well as statistical variations. In Pennsylvania, all laboratories are licensed based on their participation in periodic proficiency testing and inspection. The laboratory must analyze the blood alcohol sample spiked with an unknown amount of alcohol sent by the state and obtain results within ±10% of the expected value. In addition, the laboratory must run calibrators and at least two levels of blood controls obtained from outside manufacturers. The results obtained each day for each control are plotted against the spread of the results over the expected target value. These are called Levey-Jennings plots. It is generally accepted that these will vary by ±10 % (12,24). Some laboratories may set this variation at ±5%. At 10% variation, Daniel's BAC could be as low as 0.075% and at 5% variation, his BAC could be 0.079%.

15.5.7 Conclusions

The following conclusions can be arrived at with a reasonable degree of scientific certainty:

1. Based on Daniel's body weight, the number of beers he drank, and the time lapse between the last beer and his blood draw, his calculated BAC is below the legal limit.
2. Daniel's prescription medications slowed down the metabolism of alcohol by the liver resulting in a BAC higher than expected.
3. The blood alcohol levels determined by headspace GC are subjected to ±10% or ±5% statistical variation. Daniel's BAC might be as low as 0.075% at 10% variation or 0.079% at 5% variation.

References

1. Synergistic effects of alcohol and other drugs. http://library.thinkquest.org/12875/data/alcohol/a6.html?tql-iframe.
2. Wikipedia. Synergy. http://en.wikipedia.org/wiki/synergy.
3. DiMaio, V.J. and DiMaio, D. *Forensic Pathology*, 2nd ed. CRC Press, Boca Raton, FL, 2001.
4. Levine, B. *Principles of Forensic Toxicology*. AACC Press, Washington, D.C., 1999.
5. Zernig, G., Saria, A., Kurz, M., and O'Malley, S.S. (Eds). *Handbook of Alcoholism*. CRC Press, Boca Raton, FL, 2000.
6. Karch, S.B. *Karch's Pathology of Drug Abuse*, 3rd ed. CRC Press, Boca Raton, FL, 2001.
7. Baselt, R.C. and Cravey, R.H. *Disposition of Toxic Drugs and Chemicals in Man*, 4th ed. Chemical Toxicology Institute, Foster City, CA, 1995.
8. Micromedex® POISINDEX System.
9. Williams, R.H. and Leikin, T. Medico-legal issues and specimen collection for ethanol testing. *Lab. Med.* **30**:630–637, 1999.
10. Stowell, A.R. and Stowell, L.I. Estimation of blood alcohol concentration after social drinking. *J. Forensic Sci.* **43**:14–21, 1998.
11. Lands, W.E.M. A review of alcohol clearance in humans. *Alcohol.* **15**:147–160, 1998.
12. Burtis, C.A., Ashwood, E.R., and Burns, D.E. (Eds.) *Tietz Textbook of Clinical Chemistry and Molecular Biology*, 4th ed. W.B. Saunders Company, Philadelphia, PA, 2006.
13. Winek, C.L., Wahha, W.W., Winek Jr., C.L., and Balzer, T.W. Winek's drug and chemical blood-level data. *Forensic Sci. Int.* **122**:107–123, 2001.
14. Gillman, A.G., Goodman, L.S., Rall, T.W., and Murad, F. *Goodman and Gilman's The Pharmacological Basis of Therapeutics*. MacMillan Publishing Company, New York, 1985.

15. Ask your pharmacist. Can I drink alcohol while taking SSRI antidepressant? http://www.drugstore.com/ask/can-i-drink-alcohol-while-taking-an-ssri-anti-depressant/qxa1131, 2006.

16. DiMartini, A.F. and Rao, K.N. Elevated blood ethanol levels due to nonalcoholic beer. *J. Clin. Forensic Med.* **6**:106–108, 1999.

17. Anonymous. FDA announces new alcohol warnings for pain relievers and pain reducers. October 21, 1998. Available at http:www.fda.gov.

18. Andrejak, M., Davion, T., Gineston, J.L. et. al. Cross hepatotoxicity between non-steroidal anti-inflammatory drugs. *Br. Med. J.* **295**:180–181, 1987.

19. Law, I.P. and Knight, H. Jaundice associated with naproxen. *N. Eng. J. Med.* **295**:1201, 1976.

20. Bas, B.H. Jaundice associated with naproxen. *Lancet.* **1**:998, 1974.

21. Goodwin, J.S. and Regan, M. Cognitive dysfunction associated with naproxen and ibuprofen in the elderly. *Arthritis. Rheum.* **25**: 1013–1015, 1982.

22. Hanlon, J.T., Schmader, K.E., Landerman, L.R. et. al. Relation of prescription non-steroidal anti-inflammatory drug use to cognitive function among the community-dwelling elderly. *Ann. Epidemiol.* **7**:87–94, 1997.

23. Perkin, E. Increasing accuracy of blood alcohol analysis using headspace gas-chromatography. www.perkinelmer.com, 2008.

24. Pennsylvania code. Health and Safety. Chapter 5. Clinical Laboratories. www.pacode.com.

Breathalyzer Tests 16

In this chapter, cases are presented where the police have used breathalyzer instruments to determine a defendant's BAC. When a police officer stops a person on suspicion of DUI, he uses several techniques to determine if the person is intoxicated. He uses field sobriety tests or a preliminary breath test (PBT). PBT test instrument is a hand-held device into which the suspect is asked to blow air. The instrument gives a reading after measuring the alcohol in the breath and extrapolates it to BAC. These tests are not admissible in courts of law in several states in the United States. Nevertheless, this gives an idea to the police officer if further tests are warranted to asses a defendant's level of intoxication. He can take a suspect to the police station and subject the suspect to an approved breathalyzer instrument. Cases involving the use of different breathalyzer instruments are given.

16.1 Breathalyzer Measurements

Breath alcohol analytical instruments were developed for obtaining a suspect's blood-alcohol in a noninvasive way. These are quicker and cheaper to use than blood tests. It is much easier to ask a suspect to blow breath into an instrument rather than to obtain a blood sample, in which case the suspect needs to be taken to a hospital so that a qualified healthcare professional can draw the blood (1). As early as 1938, a device was developed to assess drunkenness and was called the drunkometer (2). Further developments led to the introduction of a variety of breathalyzer instruments (2).

16.2 Breath Alcohol Measurements and Their Extrapolation to Whole Blood Alcohol Concentration

Ethanol diffuses readily from the pulmonary arterial blood into air in the lungs. This process forms the basis of the breathalyzer tests for estimating BAC. In principle, the ethanol vapor in the breath is in equilibrium with ethanol dissolved in the water of the blood, and it is estimated that the average partition coefficient between blood and breath is 2100:1. This partition coefficient can vary between individuals. The correct partition coefficient can estimate BAC from the breath alcohol content. This estimate is reasonably accurate (1,2). However, the correct partition of an individual is not known. The instrument is checked to an average partition coefficient of 2100:1. Therefore, when BAC is estimated from a breathalyzer, the result is an estimate based on a faulty partition coefficient. For this reason, it is preferable to make conclusions on a direct measurement of alcohol from the blood. Breath alcohol measurements are subjected to various physiological variables whereas blood alcohol measurements in a certified toxicology laboratory are less prone to physiological variables. Thus, a total reliance on breath alcohol measurements could lead to erroneous conclusions. Analytical measurements by a certified laboratory usually have well-defined accuracy and precision, which are useful for indicating the reliability of measurement. There is a commonsense and scientific presumption that conviction should only occur if breath alcohol concentration obtained by the police fairly reflects the BAC, which in turn should reflect the alcohol reaching the brain, which in turn indicates the degree of alcohol-induced impairment of driving ability (3-7).

16.3   Intoxilyzer 5000

16.3.1   Legal Aspects: Presumptive DUI and
Breath Alcohol Measurements

This case is about Brian Rajas, who was stopped at a DUI checkpoint and arrested for DUI based on breath alcohol test by the Intoxilyzer 5000 instrument. He challenges the accuracy of the instrument and he contends that his BAC could not be 0.105% as he only drank two beers.

16.3.2   Medical Aspects: Accuracy of Intoxilyzer 5000

Intoxilyzer 5000 instrument measurement of breath alcohol is affected by several variables and can give falsely elevated BAC.

16.3.3   Factual Background

Mr. Brian Rajas is a Caucasian man, 41 years of age, 5 feet 7 inches tall and weighing 190 pounds on the day of his arrest for presumptive DUI. The Scott Township police stopped him at a DUI checkpoint at Ibis Road. He was driving a black 1995 Honda sedan. According to the police complaint, Brian Rajas was exhibiting signs of alcohol intoxication and was given field sobriety tests, which he failed. Consequently, he was given a breath alcohol test with the Intoxylizer 5000 instrument at 2:28 p.m. and again at 2:29 p.m. These tests gave BACs of 0.105% and 0.115%, respectively.

According to Brian, he went to a friend's house and only had two beers—one at 12:30 p.m. and another at 1:00 p.m.

16.3.4 Blood Alcohol Concentration

As stated in Chapter 13, BAC depends on several factors. In a normal healthy male weighing 200 pounds, one alcoholic drink is expected to give a BAC of 0.02%. Alcohol is also expected to dissipate from the body at the rate of 0.02% per hour (8-13). The defendant weighed 190 pounds and one alcoholic drink is expected to give a BAC of 0.021%. His BAC was measured approximately 1.5 hours after his last drink.

16.3.5 Breath Alcohol Measurements and Their Extrapolation to Whole Blood Alcohol Concentration

Ethanol diffuses readily from the pulmonary arterial blood into the air in the lungs. This process forms the basis for the breathalyzer tests for estimating BAC. In principle, the ethanol vapor in the breath is in equilibrium with ethanol dissolved in the water of the blood. Alcohol is estimated by the instrument set at an average partition coefficient of 2100:1. The correct partition coefficient can estimate BAC from the breath alcohol content (14-17). When BAC is estimated from a breathalyzer, the result is an estimate based on a faulty probability distribution. Therefore, it is preferable to make conclusions on a direct measurement of alcohol from the blood. Breath alcohol measurements are subjected to various physiological variables, whereas blood alcohol measurements are less prone to physiological variables. Thus, a total reliance on breath alcohol measurements could lead to erroneous conclusions (7).

Intoxilyzer 5000 determines ethanol by measuring the absorption of infrared radiation in breath at 3.39 mm and 3.48 mm. A third wavelength at 3.8 mm serves as a baseline for comparison with the response in the other two infrared radiation channels. A fixed blood:breath alcohol ratio is set for the instrument. Therefore, an accurate measurement of breath alcohol does not necessarily indicate a reliable estimate of BAC unless the subject's blood:breath ratio was found precisely. These ratios are known to vary widely and values ranging from 1700 to 3500 were noticed (6-9). Considering this range, if an individual has 1700:1 ratio of blood:breath alcohol, his actual BAC would be lower than the measurement obtained by breath analysis. This represents a 20% variation.

In healthy subjects, who are in the rising phase of alcohol absorption, the venous blood alcohol levels are much lower than that of the arterial blood. Consequently, breath alcohol measurements during the absorption phase are overestimated. It was found that in several subjects, alcohol does not absorb even after 90 minutes. Therefore, in these individuals, BAC could be overestimated even after 90 minutes and possibly up to 120 minutes after drinking stopped (15-20).

The defendant was operating his vehicle at 1:30 p.m. when the police stopped him. Intoxilyzer 5000 measurements were done at 2:28 p.m. and 2:29 p.m., respectively. The breathalyzer test was given 90 minutes after the defendant's last drink. Consequently, the defendant was definitely in the absorption phase of alcohol metabolism, which resulted in an overestimation of his BAC. Assuming that his Intoxilyzer 5000 measured his BAC accurately, even then his BAC would be much lower than the legal limit when he was stopped at 1:30 p.m. Since the defendant was in the absorption phase of alcohol metabolism, it is possible to calculate the defendant's BAC at various time intervals after he left his friend's house. The Intoxilyzer measurement was taken 90 minutes after his last drink. In these 90 minutes he was expected to dissipate 0.03% of alcohol from his blood. Therefore, we have to add 0.03% to the Intoxilyzer reading of 0.105%, which gives an estimated BAC of 0.135% at 2:28 p.m.

Time (h)	BAC (%)	Comments
12:30 p.m.	0	First beer
1:00 p.m.	0	Second beer, left friend's house
1:30 p.m.	0.045	Stopped by police
2:00 p.m.	0.09	
2:28 p.m.	0.135	Intoxilyzer 5000 test

The previous table illustrates the calculation of BAC at various time intervals by the Intoxilyzer 5000 measurement. When the defendant was stopped by the police, his BAC was calculated to be 0.045%. The increase in consecutive test readings of 0.105 and 0.115% by breathalyzer test suggests that the defendant was in the absorption phase of alcohol metabolism.

These results are also subject to the variation in the ratio in the individual blood/breath partition coefficient and the variation in the precision of the breathalyzer instrument (Pennsylvania regulations recognize a 0.01% variance). If the variation in the ratio of blood/breath is considered, the BAC should be 20% less than the reading of 0.105%—a reduction of 0.021%; that would be 0.084%. If the 0.015% variation in the machine is considered, it would be as low as 0.069%.

16.3.6 Conclusions

Based on the available evidence in scientific and medical literature, it can be concluded with a reasonable degree of medical and scientific certainty that:

1. The defendant was in the absorption phase of alcohol metabolism.
2. The defendant's BAC was below the legal limit when the police stopped him at 2:30 p.m.

16.4   Dragger Alcotest 7110

16.4.1   Legal Aspects: Blood Alcohol Levels Measured by Dragger Alcotest 7110

This case is about Mr. Arnold Gibbs, who was stopped by Twinpine Township police officers on suspicion of drunk driving. He was subjected to a new breathalyzer instrument—the Dragger Alcotest 7110. This instrument measured Mr. Gibbs's BAC to be 0.09%. He was charged with DUI and was arrested. Mr. Gibbs does not think he drank that many beers to get a BAC of 0.09% and challenged the accuracy of the Dragger Alcotest 7110 measurements.

16.4.2   Medical Aspects: Accuracy of Blood Alcohol Measurements by Dragger Alcotest 7110

The instrument manufacturer claims that this instrument is more accurate than are other breathalyzer instruments. However, even this instrument is influenced by several variables.

16.4.3   Factual Background

This report deals with Mr. Arnold Gibbs, a Caucasian male, 45 years of age and weighing 180 pounds. He was a plumber for Serp Heating and Cooling Company. The defendant was driving a yellow van east on Welch Road at 9:25 p.m. and allegedly crossed the double yellow lines. A police officer witnessed this and pulled the defendant over.

The police officer observed an open Miller Lite beer can in the cup holder. The officer noticed a moderate smell of alcohol. According to the police officer, the defendant failed field sobriety tests. He was taken to Twinpine Forest Township Police Station. He was administered the Dragger Alcotest 7110 at 10:05 p.m., which gave a BAC of 0.09%. Based on this result, he was charged with DUI. Mr. Gibbs admits that he drank three to four beers at home from 7:00 p.m. to 8:00 p.m. When he was about to drink his fourth beer, he got an emergency call and left home at 8:00 p.m. to attend to an emergency call. He carried the opened beer can with him and put it in the cup holder of the van. After he completed his job at about 9.15 p.m., he drank the remaining beer in the can that was left in the cup holder. He ate a light dinner at home. Mr. Gibbs is in good health and takes only Nexium.

16.4.4   Blood Alcohol Concentration

As stated previously, BAC depends on several factors. It takes approximately 60 to 90 minutes for alcohol to be completely absorbed from the GI tract and reach peak levels in the blood. In some individuals, this is known to take more than two hours. Food in the stomach is known to delay the absorption. Alcohol is metabolized by the liver and is dissipated from the blood at a rate of 0.02% per hour (8-13).

16.4.5   Calculation of BAC

It is scientifically accepted that a 150-pound man will have a BAC of 0.025% after drinking 1 oz. of 100 proof (50%) alcohol. This assumption is accurate under almost all circumstances (18).

BAC = 150 ÷ Body weight × % ethanol content ÷ 50 × ounces consumed × 0.025

Arnold weighed 180 pounds and he drank Miller Lite beer. Assuming that each beer was 12 ounces and Miller Lite beer has 4.2% alcohol, the calculated BAC would be as follows:

BAC of 1 beer = 150 ÷ 180 × 4.2 ÷ 50 × 12 × 0.025 = 0.02%

BAC of 4 beers = 0.08%

The first drink was taken at 7:00 p.m. and the third beer was taken at 7:45 p.m. He started drinking the fourth beer at 8:00 p.m., but was called for an emergency service. He carried this open beer can and put it in the cup holder in his van. He says that he drank this beer after he finished the job at 9:15 p.m. BAC due to the three beers before he left for the emergency work would be 0.06%. However, there was a time lapse of at least 1.5 hours before the police stopped him at 9:25 p.m. During this period, he was expected to dissipate 0.03% alcohol from his blood. If this were subtracted from 0.06%, the calculated BAC would be 0.03% when the police officer stopped him. The fourth beer was still being absorbed and would contribute 0.02% when the Dragger Alcotest 7110 was administered. However, since there was a time lapse of at least one additional hour, he would have dissipated 0.02% from his blood resulting in a calculated BAC of 0.03% when the breathalyzer test was administered. Yet, the Dragger Alcotest 7110 gave a BAC of 0.09%. This discrepancy may be due to underreporting beers that were consumed by Arnold Gibbs or the Dragger Alcotest 7110 overestimating his BAC.

16.4.6   Breath Alcohol Measurements and
Their Extrapolation to BAC

Ethanol diffuses readily from the pulmonary arterial blood into air in the lungs. This process forms the basis for the breathalyzer tests for estimating BAC. In principle, the ethanol vapor in the breath is in equilibrium with ethanol dissolved in blood and BAC is estimated using the average partition coefficient between blood and breath. The correct partition coefficient can indeed estimate BAC from the breath alcohol content. When BAC is estimated from a breathalyzer instrument set to a constant partition coefficient, the result is an estimate based on a faulty probability distribution. Individual variations in partition coefficient are known to occur. Therefore, it is preferable to make conclusions on a direct measurement of alcohol from blood (14-19). Breath alcohol measurements are subjected to various physiological variables, whereas blood alcohol measurements are less prone to physiological variables. Thus, a total reliance on breath alcohol measurements could lead to erroneous conclusions.

Analytical measurements by a certified laboratory usually have well-defined accuracy and precision, which are useful for indication of reliability of measurement (8-11,13,14). GC is the gold standard in the determination of blood alcohol levels. GC is not influenced by the physiological variable of the suspect. Indeed, police laboratories use GC in blood alcohol determination.

16.4.7   Dragger Alcotest 7110 Instrument

The Dragger Alcotest 7110 Instrument, even though an improvement from other breathalyzer instruments that are used by law enforcement, is still subjected to physiological variables of the suspect. A suspect blows air through the mouthpiece. When he blows sufficient air, the operator will ask the suspect to stop. The amount of air required for a valid test is 1.5 L. The Dragger Alcotest 7110 uses two different techniques to measure alcohol concentration. These are infrared absorption and electrochemical reaction. The breath air is subjected to 3.4 μm and 9.5 μm wavelength. This eliminates interference by other volatile molecules such as acetone. The machine also measures the ethanol concentration by a fuel cell. When the two results agree, the machine converts breath alcohol concentration to BAC. This machine, however, cannot determine ethanol levels in arterial blood and venous blood. Studies have shown that volume of breath air intake varies by 10%. The breath air temperature varies between individuals; therefore, to eliminate this variability the machine references to 34°C (14-19). Still, the machine cannot differentiate whether the subject is in the absorption phase or post-absorption phase. If the suspect is in the absorption phase, the machine overestimates BAC by at least 30%. Even though the manufacturer claims 5% variability, generally most of the analytical instruments have 10% variability. In addition,

Pennsylvania recognizes 10% variability in the measurements by analytical instruments. In healthy subjects in the rising phase of alcohol absorption, the venous blood alcohol levels are much lower than that of arterial blood. Consequently, breath alcohol measurements during the absorption phase are overestimated. It was found that in several subjects, alcohol does not absorb completely even after 120 minutes. Therefore, in these individuals BAC could be overestimated even after 120 minutes **(12-15)**.

16.4.8 Conclusions

Based on the published scientific literature, it can be concluded with a reasonable degree of medical and scientific certainty that:

1. Mr. Arnold Gibbs's BAC at the time the police officer stopped him and at the time the Dragger Alcotest 7110 was given was 0.03%.
2. Mr. Gibbs was in the absorption phase of alcohol metabolism and the Dragger Alcotest 7110 overestimated his BAC.
3. Mr. Gibbs's BAC was below the legal limit and he was not intoxicated when he was stopped by the police officer.

16.5 DataMaster

16.5.1 Legal Aspects: Overestimated BAC by DataMaster

This case is about Mr. Jerome Millert. The police stopped him when he was making an illegal U-turn. He was given a breath alcohol test by the DataMaster breathalyzer machine at 12:59 p.m. and 1:02 p.m. These tests gave BACs of 0.086% and 0.094%, respectively. He was charged with DUI and was arrested. He challenges the accuracy of the breathalyzer test administered to him and further contends that the number of beers he drank would not have given that high of a BAC.

16.5.2 Medical Aspects: False-Positive BAC by DataMaster Instrument

Even this breathalyzer instrument is influenced by several variables and can overestimate BAC.

16.5.3 Factual Background

This case is about Mr. Jerome Millert, a 51-year-old African American male, 5 feet 8 inches tall and weighing 180 pounds on the day of his arrest. He was arrested for DUI on May 25, 2008 at 12:18 p.m. He was stopped at the intersection of Scott Road and Lenox Drive by a police officer from Lemon Township as he was making an illegal U-turn. The police officer smelled alcohol on Jerome's breath. He was given sobriety tests by the police officer, which the defendant failed. He was given breath alcohol test by the DataMaster breathalyzer machine. Tests given at 12:59 p.m. and at 1:02 p.m. gave BACs of 0.086% and 0.094%, respectively.

Jerome admits drinking a couple of shots of tequila at a gathering for a memorial service. He volunteered to drive a woman home because she felt that she was intoxicated. He left the party at noon to drop the woman at her home. He was surprised that his BAC was 0.086% for the couple of shots of tequila consumed at the party.

16.5.4 Blood Alcohol Concentration

As stated previously, BAC depends on several factors. It takes between 60 and 90 minutes for alcohol to be completely absorbed from the GI tract and reach peak levels in the blood. In some individuals, this is known to take more than two hours. Food in the stomach is known to delay the absorption. Alcohol is metabolized by the liver and is dissipated from the blood at a rate of 0.02% in 1 hour (**8-11, 13,14**).

16.5.5 Calculation of BAC

BAC is calculated by the following formula (**18**):

BAC=150 ÷ Body weight × % ethanol content ÷ 50 × ounces consumed × 0.025

Mr. Millert weighed 180 pounds and was 5 feet 8 inches tall. He was pulled over by the police at 12:18 p.m. His BAC as determined by DataMaster at 12:59 p.m. and 1:02 p.m. was 0.086% and 0.094%, respectively. Mr. Millert thinks he drank two shots of tequila. Assuming that each shot of tequila is 1.5 oz. and the alcoholic content was 40%, his calculated BAC would be as follows:

BAC of one shot = 150 ÷ 180 × 40 ÷ 50 × 1.5 × 0.025 = 0.025%

BAC of 2 shots = 0.05%

Based on these estimates, it is possible to calculate Mr. Millert's BAC at the time he was stopped by the police. It is also assumed that he would dissipate 0.02% alcohol from blood in 1 hour. It is also assumed that the BAC determined by the DataMaster is accurate.

Time (h)	Dissipation (%)	DataMaster BAC (%)	Calculated BAC (%)	Comments
12:00 p.m.	0	0	0	Left the party
12:15 p.m.	0.005	0.215	0.265	Stopped by police
12:30 p.m.	0.01	0.043	0.053	
12:45 p.m.	0.015	0.0645	0.0795	
12:59 p.m.	0.02	0.086	0.108	DataMaster test

Based on these calculations, Mr. Jerome Millert probably drank three shots of tequila. Two consecutive readings at 3 minutes apart by the instrument gave readings of 0.086% and 0.094%. These readings suggest that Mr. Jerome Millert was in the absorption phase of alcohol metabolism. From the previous table, his calculated BAC when the police stopped him was below the legal limit. If it is argued that it is the statistical variation by the machine, then this variability comes to about 9.3%. In such a case, his calculated BAC with 9.3% variation could be as low as 0.078%. This is indeed below the legal limit. All the breathalyzer instruments are known to overestimate BAC when a subject is in the absorption phase of alcohol metabolism.

16.5.6 Breath Alcohol Measurements and Their Extrapolation to BAC

Ethanol diffuses readily from the pulmonary arterial blood into air in the lungs. This process forms the basis for the breathalyzer tests for estimating BAC. In principle, ethanol vapors in the breath are in equilibrium with ethanol dissolved in the water of the blood and it is estimated that the average partition coefficient between blood and breath is 2100:1. The correct partition coefficient can estimate BAC from the breath alcohol content (14-17). When BAC is estimated from a breathalyzer, the result is an estimate based on a faulty probability distribution. Therefore, it is preferable to make conclusions on a direct measurement of alcohol from the blood (17). Breath alcohol measurements are subjected to various physiological variables, whereas blood alcohol measurements are less prone to physiological variables. Thus, a total reliance on breath alcohol measurements could lead to erroneous conclusions (17).

Analytical measurements by a certified laboratory usually have well-defined accuracy and precision, which are useful for indicating the reliability of measurement. There is a commonsense and scientific presumption that conviction should only occur if BAC obtained by the police fairly reflects the BAC, which in turn should reflect the alcohol reaching the brain, which in turn indicates the degree of acute alcohol-induced impairment of driving ability (8-13).

Breathalyzer instruments, in general, determine ethanol by measuring the absorption of infrared radiation. A fixed blood breath alcohol ratio such as 2100:1 is set for the instrument. Therefore, a reliable measurement of breath alcohol does not necessarily indicate a reliable estimate of BAC unless the subject's blood/breath ratio was found precisely. These ratios are known to vary widely and values ranging from 1700 to 3500 were noticed (15). Considering this range, if an individual has 1700:1 ratio of blood to breath alcohol, his actual BAC would be lower than the measurement obtained by breath analysis. This represents a 20% variation.

In healthy subjects in the rising phase of alcohol absorption, the venous blood alcohol levels are much lower than the levels of the arterial blood. Consequently, breath alcohol measurements during the absorption phase are overestimated. It was found that in several subjects, alcohol does not absorb even after 90 minutes. Therefore, in these individuals, BAC could be overestimated even after 90 minutes and possibly up to 120 minutes after drinking stopped (14-17).

16.5.7   DataMaster

National Patent Analytical Systems Inc., Mansfield, Ohio, manufactures this breathalyzer instrument. The DataMaster is used in several states in this country. However, the scientific community believes that breathalyzers tests, in general, are less accurate to determine blood alcohol levels. With DataMaster, the subjects are asked to blow a deep breath into the mouthpiece of the instrument. Consecutive breath samples provided by the subjects vary widely, resulting in variation in the readings provided by the instrument. Pennsylvania allows 10% variation by the instrument. Mouth alcohol affects readings by this instrument. Blood:breath alcohol ratio is set with the instrument at 2100:1. This ratio is known to vary as low as 1700:1 and as high as 3500:1 (15). This affects the BAC determined by the machine because it is difficult to know the blood:breath ratio of any given individual. As with other breathalyzer instruments, the BAC determined by the machine is falsely elevated if a subject is in the absorption phase of alcohol metabolism.

16.5.8   Conclusions

Based on the available evidence, it is concluded with a reasonable degree of medical and scientific certainty that:

1. Mr. Jerome Millert was in the absorption phase of alcohol metabolism and the breathalyzer machine overestimated his BAC.

2. Even when it is assumed that that DataMaster determined his BAC levels accurately, his actual BAC at the time he was stopped by the police was below the legal limit.
3. Two consecutive readings by the DataMaster machine showed 9.3% variation. If this variation is taken into consideration, his BAC could be 0.078%, which is below the legal limit.

References

1. CMI Inc. Breath alcohol testing basics. Why breath alcohol analysis? http://www.alcoholtest.com/index.php.
2. Wikipedia. Breathalyzer. http://en.wikipedia.org/wiki/Breathalyzer.
3. Dubowski, K.M. Absorption, distribution and elimination of alcohol: highway safety aspects. *J. Studies Alcohol Suppl.* **10**:98–107, 1985.
4. Jones, A.W. and Anderson, L. Variability of blood/breath ratio in drinking drivers. *J. Forensic Sci.* **41**:916–921, 1996.
5. Simpson, G. Accuracy and precision of breath-alcohol measurements for a random subject in post-absorptive state. *Clin. Chem.* **33**:261–268, 1987.
6. Trafford, D.J.H. and Makin, H.L.J. Breath-alcohol concentration may not always reflect the concentration of alcohol in blood. *J. Anal. Toxicol.* **18**:225–228, 1994.
7. Jones, A.W., Beylich, K.M., Bjorneboe, A., Ingum, J., and Morland, J. Measuring ethanol in blood and breath for legal purposes: variability between laboratories and between breath test instruments. *Clin. Chem.* **38**:743–747, 1992.
8. Williams, R.H. and Leikin, J.B. Medico-legal issues and specimen collection for ethanol testing. *Lab. Med.* **30**:630–637, 1999.
9. Stowell, A.R. and Stowell, L.I. Estimation of blood alcohol concentration after social drinking. *J. Forensic Sci.* **43**:114–121, 1998.
10. Lands, W.E.M. A review of alcohol clearance in humans. *Alcohol* **15**:147–160, 1997.
11. Begleiter, H. and Kissin, B. *The Pharmacology of Alcohol and Alcohol Dependence.* Oxford University Press, New York, 1996, 24–26.
12. DiMaio, V.J., and DiMaio, D. *Forensic Pathology*, 2nd ed. CRC Press, Boca Raton, FL, 2001.
13. Levine, B. *Principles of Forensic Toxicology.* AACC Press, Washington, D.C., 1999.
14. Dubowski, K.M. Absorption, distribution and elimination of alcohol: highway safety aspects. *J. Studies Alcohol Suppl.* **10**:98–107, 1985.
15. Jones, A.W. and Anderson, L. Variability of blood/breath ratio in drinking drivers. *J. Forensic Sci.* **41**:916–921, 1996.
16. Simpson, G. Accuracy and precision of breath-alcohol measurements for a random subject in post-absorptive state. *Clin. Chem.* **33**:261–268, 1987.
17. Trafford, D.J.H. and Makin, H.L.J. Breath-alcohol concentration may not always reflect the concentration of alcohol in blood. *J. Anal. Toxicol.* **18**:225–228, 1994.
18. Karch, S.B. *Karch's Pathology of Drug Abuse*, 3rd ed. CRC Press, Boca Raton, FL, 2001.
19. Beck, C.M. and Flack, H.J. Development of a system for real time breath alcohol analysis. www.druglibrary.org/schaffer/misc/driving/s30p16.htm 2007.

Dram Shop Liability 17

In this chapter, several interesting cases that come under the dram shop liability laws (laws that deal with the responsibility of the bar and tavern owners who serve alcohol to the public) are presented.

Alcoholic dram shop or dramshop is a term that is used to describe a bar, tavern, or establishment that serves alcohol by a small unit of liquid. Our court system recognizes an injured party's right to pursue the seller of alcohol for damages caused by the acts of an injured adult customer (1). Under dram shop liability law, a party injured by an intoxicated person can sue the establishment that contributed to that person's intoxication. It is interesting to note that in Texas, minors can sue the drinking establishment for their own injuries sustained while intoxicated (2). Generally, dram shop laws establish the liability of establishments rising out of selling alcohol to visibly intoxicated persons or minors who subsequently cause damage to third parties. These laws have drawn criticism as they downplay the role of personal responsibility (3).

In addition to drunken driving accidents causing injuries and fatalities, alcohol also contributes to violent crimes. The law recognizes that bars have an obligation to their customers as well as the public to prevent alcohol-induced intoxication resulting in motor vehicle accidents. Bar owners have an obligation to cut off those who drink too much. They are expected to provide adequate security (4,5).

17.1 Alcohol, Carbon Monoxide, and Death of a Female Motorist

17.1.1 Legal Aspects: Responsibility of the Bar

This case is about Mary Haddar, a Caucasian female, 40 years of age, who was found unconscious due to alcohol intoxication and carbon monoxide poisoning in her car. She was transported to the hospital where she died despite the best efforts of the doctors to revive her. Her two sons are suing the bar where she drank alleging that their mother died because of the negligence of the bar for serving her alcohol even though she was intoxicated.

17.1.2 Medical Aspects: Alcohol Intoxication and Carbon Monoxide Poisoning

Because of alcohol intoxication, Mary became lethargic and fell asleep at the wheel. Her car was old and had a faulty exhaust system that emitted carbon monoxide into the car. With the widows rolled up, the carbon monoxide had nowhere to go. This resulted in Mary becoming unconscious.

17.1.3 Factual Background

Mary Haddar was a Caucasian female, 40 years of age, and weighed 150 pounds. She was thrice divorced and had two teenage sons. She was found unconscious in a parking lot at 8:00 a.m. on February 11, 1999. An ambulance transported her to the hospital. Despite their best efforts at the emergency room, Mary died. The unfortunate demise of this apparently healthy individual could have been easily prevented.

Mary went to the Tiger's Bar at approximately 1:00 p.m. on February 10, 1999 and left the bar at 3:00 a.m. the next day. Several of her friends and acquaintances stated that she was at the bar for 14 to 15 hours and was drinking draft beer all night. Some acquaintances became concerned as they thought that Mary drank nearly 20 beers. They asked the bartender to stop serving Mary beer. According to the eyewitness account, Mary left the bar at 3:00 a.m. Mary's car was found parked at the parking lot of Tiger's Bar. A tow truck was called in and the tow truck driver found Mary unconscious lying on the front seat of her car, with the engine running, lights and wipers on at 8:00 p.m. An ambulance was called and Mary was transported to Xinna Memorial Hospital. She was pronounced dead at the emergency room. The death was ruled due to alcohol intoxication and carbon monoxide poisoning.

17.1.4 Alcohol Intoxication

Blood alcohol levels depend on the weight of the person, age, gender, health, food in the stomach, medications, and co-abuse of drugs. Ethanol is water-soluble and is absorbed rapidly into the body within 30 to 90 minutes. Women may have less gastric alcohol dehydrogenase activity than men, which may explain why women generally have higher peak ethanol levels and may have higher toxic effects of ethanol than men (6). One alcoholic beverage results in a level of 0.02% in blood in a 200-pound man. Alcohol levels are dissipated from blood at a rate of 0.02% per hour. These assumptions are applicable to men but are not quite accurate for women. Assuming that a person is in normal health, it is possible to calculate the number of drinks a person had and the toxicity associated with it provided the blood alcohol levels and the time frame in which the person drank are known (7,8). Mary was 150 pounds, and was seen drinking draft beer from the time she entered the bar at 1:00 p.m. on February 10, 1999. Mary left the bar at 3:00 a.m. on February 11, 1999. Therefore, the deceased spent nearly 14 hours at the bar. The serum alcohol levels were determined at the hospital at 9:00 a.m. by GC and it can be assumed that blood was drawn immediately on admission at 8:50 a.m. Her serum alcohol level was 0.26% which works out to be 0.24% in whole blood applying a conversion factor of 1.1 (9,10). Her blood pH was 6.72, with very low serum bicarbonate. This was consistent with her being acidotic due to alcohol intoxication. There was a time lapse of 6 hours from the time she left the bar to the time of her blood draw. Assuming that she dissipated 0.02% alcohol from her blood, she would have metabolized 0.12% when she left the bar at 3:00. If this is added to the blood alcohol level of 0.24% at the time of the blood draw, her calculated blood alcohol levels should be 0.36%. She weighed 150 pounds and one drink was expected to give a blood alcohol level of 0.026%. As stated earlier, these calculations are only approximations, as females tend to have higher blood alcohol levels and tend to dissipate at a slower rate than men do. To get to an expected level of 0.36%, the deceased must have consumed at least 15 beers. This corroborates the eyewitness account of Sue McDavitt, who felt that the deceased drank at least 20 beers. Veronica, another eyewitness, as well as others at the bar thought that the bartender should have stopped Mary earlier from purchasing additional beers.

The deceased had blood alcohol level that was nearly four times the legal limit at the time of her hospitalization. Alcohol, being a drug, has known and observable signs and measurable effects on many physiological activities of the body (9,10). Alcohol has effects on the CNS and impairs several motor and physiological responses. This impairment occurs in virtually most of the individuals at or above 80 mg/dL. That is why the legal limit of blood alcohol level was set at 80 mg/dL. Therefore, it is reasonable to conclude that the deceased exhibited visible signs of intoxication at the bar.

It is also possible to back-calculate with reasonable scientific certainty her blood alcohol levels at various time intervals by adding alcohol dissipated from her blood to 0.24, the alcohol levels at blood draw.

Time (h)	Alcohol Dissipated (%)	Calculated BAC (%)	Comments
3:00 a.m.	0.12	0.36	Left the bar
4:00 a.m.	0.10	0.34	
5:00 a.m.	0.08	0.32	
6:00 a.m.	0.06	0.30	
7:00 a.m.	0.04	0.28	
8:00 a.m.	0.02	0.26	
9:00 a.m.	0	0.24	Blood draw

The above calculations show that the blood alcohol of the deceased reached extremely high toxic levels and fatalities are known to occur at 400 mg/dL. At these levels, the bartender should have easily noticed the symptoms of intoxication in Mary. The bar was negligent in serving alcohol to the deceased. When Mary left the bar, her blood alcohol levels were so high it made her lethargic and sleepy (**9,10**).

17.1.5 Conclusions

As stated in the death certificate, the deceased had alcohol intoxication, which contributed to her unconsciousness, and subsequently she was exposed to carbon monoxide from her car. With a reasonable degree of scientific certainty, it can be concluded that:

1. Mary exhibited symptoms of alcohol intoxication to everyone at the bar.
2. The bartender could have easily prevented this unfortunate death by shutting Mary off from buying unlimited alcoholic beverages.
3. The bar was negligent in not paying attention to Mary's symptoms of intoxication and providing help to her.

17.2 Alcohol Intoxication, Backed up Car, Fatal Drop down a Hill, and Death

17.2.1 Legal Aspects: Intoxicated Driver Backed down a Hill to His Death

This case is about Mr. John Doe, who died due to alcohol intoxication. He was a white male, 52 years of age, and an unemployed steelworker who lived with his mother. He was divorced and had three children who do not live with him. On the day of the incident, John visited River Shore Bar and Grill. He parked his car in the parking lot by the side of the bar and had a few drinks before leaving. He backed up his car, crashed into a fence, and plunged approximately 80 feet into a valley below the bar. He was found dead in his car. His family brought a civil suit against the bar and contended that the bartender was irresponsible for serving him drinks even when he was already intoxicated and thus caused his death.

17.2.2 Medical Aspects: Alcohol Induced Intoxication

The bartender has the right to refuse to serve drinks if a customer is drunk or if the bartender suspects that the customer has already had too many drinks. Chronic alcoholics do not show visual symptoms of inebriation. John Doe's blood alcohol level was found to be several times higher than the legal limit. Alcohol causes CNS depression, loss of critical judgment, impairment of depth perception, and comprehension. A chronic alcoholic may also suffer decreased sensory response, increased reaction times, loss of visual acuity, loss of peripheral vision, and mental confusion.

17.2.3   Factual Background

John Doe was a Caucasian male, 52 years of age, weighed 205 pounds, and was 5 feet 10 inches tall. He came to the River Shore Bar and Grill at approximately 6:00 p.m. He drank six cans of beer and left the bar thereafter. Sometime later, his pickup truck was discovered having plunged 80 feet down a hill and landed on its roof by the side of the railroad tracks. Mr. John Doe was found dead in his car.

From police reports and transcripts of interviews conducted with his friends and acquaintances at the bar, the events leading to the accident can be reconstructed as follows. John Doe was living with his mother. He was divorced, and was an unemployed steelworker. According to his friends, he was a chronic alcoholic. He usually frequented the bars nearby.

He was a good customer to River Shore Bar and Grill and was known to drink all types of alcohol. He kept his lawn, house, and car neat and clean. On the day of the accident, there was some indication that he came into the bar earlier in the afternoon, had few drinks, and then left. He came in again at approximately 5:30 p.m. One of his friends who came into the bar later says that he saw John Doe's car parked in the parking lot by the side of the bar with the backside toward the fence below which there was a drop of 80 to 100 feet down a hill. Mr. Doe had a few more drinks, ordered a six-pack of beer, and left the bar at approximately 6:00 p.m.

According to the police investigative reports, he drove his car backward into a white fence, as evidenced by paint marks on the rear bumper of the car, plunged 80 feet down a hill, and landed by the side of the railroad tracks. The car landed on its roof and sustained extensive damage. The train engineers noticed the car at approximately 6:45 p.m. The police, the fire department, and the paramedics arrived shortly thereafter. Mr. Doe was found trapped in the car. He was pronounced dead at the scene at 7:10 p.m.

The police safety inspection revealed that the car had no mechanical problems and that there was rearward movement of the engine and transmission, confirming the suspicion of the police that Mr. Doe drove his car backward and went over the hill. A partially consumed cigarette was found in his car near his fingertips.

Bill Bowser, MD conducted a thorough autopsy. He concluded that Mr. Doe died of blunt force trauma to the head and trunk when his car went through the parking lot fence and wound up resting on the roof of his car.

Microscopic analysis of the liver showed fatty changes, which confirmed that Mr. Doe was a chronic alcoholic. Toxicology analysis of blood, urine, and the vitreous fluid were performed at the county crime laboratory. All the body fluids examined were negative for drugs of abuse. The alcohol was determined by GC. He had 0.25% alcohol in his blood, 0.26% in urine, and 0.21% in vitreous fluid. These results suggested that Mr. Doe's blood alcohol was more than three times higher than the legal limit. He was definitely intoxicated and was unfit to drive a vehicle.

17.2.4   Alcohol Intoxication

Alcohol is a water-soluble compound that is rapidly absorbed from the GI tract within 30 to 60 minutes. It distributes to several body compartments and blood levels correlate with the toxicity of alcohol (7,10,11). A blood alcohol level of 0.08% is the legal limit in Pennsylvania. Mr. Doe's alcohol levels in urine, bile, and vitreous fluid are consistent with his blood alcohol level of 0.25%. At these blood alcohol levels, Mr. Doe suffered CNS depression, loss of critical judgment, impairment of depth perception, and loss of comprehension. He also suffered decreased sensory response, increased reaction times, reduced visual acuity, reduced peripheral vision, and mental confusion (10, 11).

As stated earlier, Mr. Doe was a chronic alcoholic. Mr. Doe went to the bar a couple of times on that day. Thus, it is possible that the bartender present in the afternoon might not have been there in the evening. It is not possible to know the actual number of drinks Mr. Doe had that day. He was a chronic alcoholic and an experienced drinker. It is known that chronic alcoholics do not show the visual symptoms of inebriation to which inexperienced drinkers are subject. He weighed 200 pounds and one alcoholic drink would result in a blood alcohol level of 0.02%. He was expected to dissipate 0.02% alcohol in 1 hour (1-3). Therefore, to get a residual level of 0.25% of blood alcohol, Mr. Doe must have consumed a large quantity of alcohol.

17.2.5   Conclusions

Based on the available evidence, it can be concluded with a reasonable degree of scientific certainty that:

1. Mr. John Doe was a chronic alcoholic who went to the bar at different times in the day and had an unknown number of drinks, which resulted in residual blood alcohol levels of 0.025%.
2. Mr. Doe suffered CNS depression, loss of critical judgment, impairment of depth perception and comprehension, decreased sensory

response, increased reaction times, loss of visual acuity, loss of peripheral vision, and resultant mental confusion.

3. Mr. Doe was responsible for driving the car backward, hitting the fence, and plunging 80 feet over a hill to his death.

17.3   Two-Car Collision, Multiple Traumas

17.3.1   Legal Aspects: Alcohol, Two-Car Collision, and Injuries

This case deals with a serious accident involving two automobiles on May 16, 1998 at 10:12 p.m. Howard was driving his pickup truck southbound on Route 296 at the same time that Brian was driving his car northbound. Brian lost control of his car, swerved into the southbound lane, and hit the oncoming pickup truck. This accident resulted in multiple traumas and permanent injuries to Howard. Howard alleges that Brian was intoxicated and unfit to drive a car. He sued the bar for failing to notice the visible signs of intoxication and to stop Brian from drinking.

17.3.2   Medical Aspects: Alcohol Intoxication

The police arrived at the accident scene at 10:19 p.m. and noticed that Brian was visibly intoxicated with alcoholic breath and glassy and bloodshot eyes. He had lack of coordination and exhibited slurred speech. The police officer obtained Brian's blood. The State Police Regional Crime Laboratory subsequently determined the BAC to be 0.14%.

17.3.3   Factual Background

This case deals with an accident involving two automobiles on May 16, 1998 at 10:12 p.m. Howard, a white male, 18 years of age, was traveling in his pickup truck, southbound on Route 296 in the town of Trenton. At the same time, Brian was driving his car in the opposite lane. Brian lost control of his car, swerved into the southbound lane, and hit Howard's pickup truck. Brian is a white male, 59 years of age, 5 feet 10 inches tall and weighing 180 pounds. The accident resulted in multiple traumas, broken bones, and permanent injuries to Howard.

The police arrived at the accident scene at 10:19 p.m. and noticed that Brian was visibly intoxicated and exhibited alcoholic breath, and glassy and bloodshot eyes. He exhibited a lack of coordination and had slurred speech. The police officer took him to an area hospital and a blood sample was drawn at 12:36 a.m. on May 17, 1998. His BAC was found to be 0.14%.

Brian went to Cheers Club at 2:30 p.m. and drank two beers. From there he went to Canadian Lagoon Bar in Bethel at 4:00 p.m. He started drinking beers and claims that he had five beers while playing cards with other people. He contends that his last beer was at 9:00 p.m. The card game broke up when the bar was ready to close at 10:00 p.m. He left the bar at 10:00 p.m., got into his car, and started driving on Route PA 296. A few minutes later, he lost control of his car and hit the oncoming pickup truck driven by Howard.

17.3.4 Brian's Blood Alcohol Levels

Brian claims that his last drink was at 9:00 p.m. and the blood draw was at 12:36 a.m., a time lapse of 3 hours and 36 minutes. Since he was expected to dissipate 0.02% of alcohol per hour (7,10), he would have dissipated 0.07% of alcohol from his blood. The crime laboratory determined his BAC to be 0.14% in his blood drawn at 12:36 a.m. Therefore, 0.07% alcohol dissipated from his blood needs to be added to 0.14%, the BAC found at the time of the blood draw, which results in a BAC of 0.21%. Based on the time of his last drink, his BAC can be calculated at various time intervals including Brian's presence in the bar as well as at the time of accident and the time of his blood draw. The calculations are as follows:

Time (h)	BAC (%)	Comments
8:00 p.m.	0.23	
9:00 p.m.	0.21	Last drink
10:00 p.m.	0.19	
10:15 p.m.	0.185	Accident
11:00 p.m.	0.17	
12:00 a.m.	0.15	
12:36 a.m.	0.14	Blood draw

Since Brian weighed 180 pounds, one alcoholic drink was expected to give a BAC of 0.022%. To get a BAC of 0.21 prior to his last drink, he would have had to consume at least 9 to 10 drinks. This is reasonable because he was at the bar from 4:00 p.m. until the bar closed at 10:00 p.m. It is realistic to think that in 5 hours he could have easily consumed 10 drinks.

Brian was severely intoxicated with alcohol. A BAC of 0.21% would result in disorientation, mental confusion, dizziness, lack of coordination, staggering, and slurred speech (10,12). At this BAC, Brian was clearly unfit to drive.

The police officer noticed these visible signs of intoxication a few minutes after Brian left the bar and yet the bartender failed to notice these signs of intoxication. According to the police officer, Brian failed field sobriety tests a few minutes after he left the bar. These observations underscore the fact that

Brian was severely intoxicated prior to his last drink at the bar (**10-12**). The bartender should not have served drinks to Brian because he was showing signs of alcohol intoxication.

17.3.5   Conclusions

1. Brian was highly intoxicated due to alcohol even before his last drink at 9:00 p.m. at the bar.
2. At this level of intoxication, he would have exhibited the symptoms of alcohol intoxication. An experienced bartender should not have missed the signs of intoxication. The bartender was irresponsible to serve alcoholic drinks to a person when he was intoxicated.
3. The accident was due to Brian's alcohol intoxication as he was unfit to drive a motor vehicle when he left the bar.

17.4   Alcohol, Marijuana, and Death of a Bicyclist

17.4.1   Legal Aspects: Presumptive DUI, Fatal Accident, and Death

This case is about the death of a bicyclist, Mr. Chuck Edwards, due to head-on collision by a pickup truck driven by Mr. Jim Johnson and with Mr. Bob Baskey as his passenger.

The wife of Mr. Edwards is suing the insurance company of Jim Johnson and HoHo bar.

17.4.2   Medical Aspects: Synergistic Toxicity of Alcohol and Marijuana

It is well established that alcohol can cause intoxication of the driver of a motor vehicle. This is further enhanced by the simultaneous use of marijuana.

17.4.3   Factual Background

This fatal accident happened during the early morning hours of July 31, 2000. It appears that Mr. Chuck Edwards was riding his bicycle south on Route 99. A 1966 Dodge Ram pickup truck driven by Mr. Jim Johnson with Mr. Bob Baskey as the passenger, going north on Route 99, struck the bicyclist head-on. Mr. Edwards was thrown off of his bicycle, struck the pickup truck, and landed in a ditch on the east side of the road. Mr. Johnson and his passenger fled the scene leaving Mr. Edwards with multiple injuries to die. The fire department located the body at 6:10 a.m. and the coroner pronounced him dead at the scene at 7:10 a.m.

The driver of the pickup truck, Mr. Johnson is a Caucasian male, 5 feet 11 inches tall and weighing 200 pounds on the day of the accident. He came back from work at 1:00 p.m. and drank four beers in a tavern. He went to a pub at 3:00 p.m. and drank two beers. He went to a Pizza Hut at 4:30 p.m. and drank a pitcher of beer (equivalent to four beers) and ate pizza. He went home at 6:00 p.m. and stayed there for an hour. He then went to the apartment of his friend, Mr. Hunter, at 7:00 p.m. At 8:00 p.m. he borrowed Mr. Hunter's pickup truck and drove 12 miles to Reion City and arrived at HoHo Bar at 8:30 p.m. He then started drinking several more beers and alcoholic beverages, including White Russians. He smoked marijuana and continued drinking more alcoholic beverages until he left the bar at 1:00 a.m. with Mr. Baskey as his passenger. It became evident during the police investigation that Vicki and Steven Dinado were at HoHo Bar from 9:30 p.m. to 11:30 p.m. They observed that Mr. Johnson was visibly intoxicated and yet he was being served alcoholic beverages by the bartenders. They noted that Mr. Johnson had difficulty standing up and was losing his balance. He was stumbling. He had blood-shot eyes and experienced difficulty focusing his eyesight. He appeared close to passing out. He left the bar with Mr. Baskey at approximately 1:00 a.m. and drove the pickup truck on the back roads to avoid the police. He struck Mr. Edwards at 1:30 a.m., resulting in his multiple traumas and death. After fleeing the scene, Mr. Johnson went to Mr. Hunter's apartment where the police picked him up, took him to the hospital, and had his blood drawn at 8:11 a.m. The blood was analyzed for alcohol by a headspace GC at the state police laboratory at Pearie. His BAC was 0.069%.

17.4.4   Blood Alcohol Concentration

As stated before, BAC depends on several factors including the number of alcoholic beverages consumed, their alcoholic content, and the time lapse between the time at which the last drink was consumed and time at which blood was drawn. In addition, the age, gender of a person, body weight, medications, health, and co-abuse of drugs also influence BAC. A normal healthy 200-pound man is expected to reach a BAC of 20 mg/dl or 0.02% with one alcoholic drink. Alcohol is dissipated from blood at a rate of 0.02% per hour (7,10-12). Based on the available evidence, the level of intoxication of the defendant needs to be established.

Based on the evidence from the deposition testimony of Vicki and Steven Dinado, the pickup truck driver, Jim Johnson, is a confirmed chronic alcoholic who co-abuses marijuana with alcohol. Mr. Johnson started drinking several alcoholic beverages at 1:30 p.m. on July 30, 2000. He continued to drink in HoHo Bar until he left at 1:00 a.m. on July 31, 2000 with his passenger

Mr. Baskey. He admitted that he was severely intoxicated, he smoked marijuana, and he drove on back roads to avoid the police. The deposition testimony of Vicki and Steven Dinado indicated that Mr. Johnson was present at
the HoHo Bar from 9:30 p.m. to 11:30 p.m. According to them, Mr. Johnson
was visibly intoxicated and yet he was continued to be served alcoholic beverages by the bartenders. Mr. Johnson was unsteady on his feet, staggering, losing his balance, and had watery and bloodshot eyes. All of these symptoms are
consistent with severe alcohol intoxication (**7,10-12**). The BAC of Mr. Johnson
determined at 8:10 a.m. was 0.069%. Based on the available evidence, it is possible to determine the following:

1. BAC of Mr. Johnson at the time of the accident.
2. Level of Mr. Johnson's intoxication.
3. Mr. Johnson's BAC between the hours of 9:30 p.m. and 11:30 p.m.
   when Vicki and Steven Dinado observed him.
4. Mr. Johnson's BAC when he left the HoHo bar at 1:00 a.m.

Since alcohol dissipates from blood at a rate of 0.02% per hour, it is possible to calculate Mr. Johnson's BAC at various time intervals as follows:

Date	Time (h)	BAC (%)	Comments
7/30/2000	8:30 p.m.	0.10	Arrived at HoHo Bar
	9:00 p.m.	0.16	
	10:00 p.m.	0.27	
	11:00 p.m.	0.25	
	12:00 a.m.	0.25	
7/31/2000	1:00 a.m.	0.21	Left HoHo Bar
	1:30 a.m.	0.20	Accident
	2:00 a.m.	0.19	
	3:00 a.m.	0.17	
	4:00 a.m.	0.15	
	5:00 a.m.	0.13	
	6:00 a.m.	0.11	
	7:00 a.m.	0.09	
	8:00 a.m	0.07	
	8:10 a.m.	0.069	

Mr. Johnson started drinking alcohol in the afternoon on July 30, 2000.
The number of beers was considerable and the resulting BAC at any given time
would be influenced by the alcoholic intake and its dissipation from blood. He
entered the HoHo Bar at approximately 8:30 p.m. and his BAC on his arrival
at the HoHo Bar is estimated to be around 0.1%. He started drinking beer and

White Russians and by 10:00 p.m., his BAC was estimated to be 0.27%. This is consistent with the observations made by other witnesses at the bar. When Mr. Johnson left the bar, his BAC was expected to be 0.21% and at the time of accident, his BAC was 0.2%, twice the legal limit. At these blood alcohol levels, a person would be expected to show loss of motor coordination, loss of visual acuity, disorientation, mental confusion, staggering, dizziness, decreased sensory response, and increased reaction times. Clearly, Mr. Johnson was incapable of driving a motor vehicle, and the accident was due to his irresponsible behavior. The death of Mr. Edwards was unnecessary.

17.4.5   Conclusions

It can be concluded with a reasonable degree of scientific certainty that:

1. Mr. Johnson was highly intoxicated with alcohol and marijuana. His BAC at the time of the fatal accident was twice the legal limit and as such was unfit to drive a motor vehicle.
2. When Mr. Johnson arrived at the HoHo Bar, he was legally intoxicated. He showed visible signs of alcohol intoxication as corroborated by the sworn testimony of the patrons present at the bar. The HoHo Bar was irresponsible in serving alcoholic drinks to Mr. Johnson, who was exhibiting symptoms of severe alcohol intoxication.

17.5   DUI, Two-Car Collision, and Vehicular Homicide

17.5.1   Legal Aspects: DUI and Vehicular Homicide

This case is about a two-car collision resulting in the death of Mr. Rob Miller. The police arrested Mr. Bruce Bettis for DUI and vehicular homicide. Mr. Bettis was subsequently convicted for this crime. Mrs. Betty Miller brought a civil lawsuit for monetary compensation for the death of her husband against the Kaloha Bar for their negligence in serving alcohol to Mr. Bettis even when he was intoxicated. On the other hand, the bar contends that Mr. Bettis was a chronic alcoholic who did not show visual signs of intoxication. Therefore, they are not responsible for the death of Mr. Miller.

17.5.2   Medical Aspects: Synergistic Toxicity of Prozac and Alcohol

Patients taking Prozac are advised not to drink alcohol and operate a motor vehicle because this drug interferes with cognitive functions and may impair judgment and motor skills. Even if a chronic alcoholic is able to mask the visual signs of intoxication from a bartender and a police officer, he or she is physiologically subjected to the intoxicating effects of alcohol.

17.5.3   Factual Background

This report is about a two-car collision resulting in multiple injuries to both drivers. The driver of one of the cars subsequently died. The accident happened on January 6, 2001. The details of the accident are as follows.

Bruce Bettis is a Caucasian male, 52 years of age and weighing 165 pounds on the day of the accident. He was coming from Red Rose Bar and Grill on Limestone Road and proceeded on River Road to go home. He was driving a KIA 1999 sedan. He crossed the center double yellow lines and hit a Pontiac station wagon operated by Rob Miller. Mr. Miller was a Caucasian male, 74 years of age, at the time of the accident. Both drivers were trapped in their vehicles and were extricated by a Rolling Hills Rescue Unit. Mr. Bettis and Mr. Miller were injured and were transported to St. Joseph Hospital. Mr. Miller was pronounced dead on January 8, 2001 at 5:00 a.m. According to the coroner, the immediate cause of death was pneumonia due to paraplegia, due to blunt force trauma of the head and neck.

The police arrived at the accident scene within a few minutes of the accident. According to the police officer, Mr. Bettis had a faint alcoholic breath, normal speech, no unusual behavior, and a cooperative attitude. When Mr. Bettis was brought to the hospital, the police obtained three vials of blood for alcohol testing by the County Crime Laboratory. The blood was drawn at 2:05. Analysis gave a BAC of 0.23%. After Mr. Miller's death, Mr. Bettis was convicted in the criminal case and is serving a 3- to 6-year sentence in a state correctional institution.

On January 6, 2001, Mr. Bettis consumed alcoholic beverages at the Kaloha Bar from 7:30 a.m. to approximately noon. He consumed these drinks at an even and steady pace for 4.5 hours. He does not remember the number of drinks he consumed. He did not eat at the bar. Thus, he drank these alcoholic beverages on an empty stomach. Mr. Bettis takes 20 mg of Prozac once a day in the morning and 50 mg of trazodone, as needed for sleep. He also takes Alka-Seltzer. He took 20 mg of Prozac in the morning before going to the bar. He was playing video slot machines. The accident happened after he left the bar probably around 12:30 p.m. Mr. Bettis has a history of alcohol abuse and can be classified as a chronic alcoholic.

17.5.4   Blood Alcohol Concentration

In a normal healthy man, weighing 200 pounds, one alcoholic drink is expected to give a BAC of 0.02%. Alcohol is also dissipated at a rate of 0.02% per hour (**7,10-12**). Mr. Bettis weighed 165 pounds. Therefore, one alcoholic drink is expected to give a BAC of 0.024%. His blood was drawn at 2:04 p.m. at which time his BAC was 0.23%. The accident happened at approximately 12:30 p.m., a time lapse of 1.5 hours between the accident and the blood draw. Therefore, he must have dissipated 0.03% of blood alcohol, which needs to be added to 0.23%. This comes to 0.26% BAC at the time of the accident. To get this BAC Mr. Bettis must have consumed between 11 and 12 drinks. This is a reasonable estimate as it is possible to consume this many drinks from the time he entered the bar at 7:30 a.m. to the time he left at 12:30 p.m. If we assume that he consumed 12 drinks at a steady rate in approximately 5 hours, it is possible to calculate his expected BAC at various time intervals to the time of his blood draw at 2:04 p.m.

Time (h)	Drinks Consumed	Expected BAC (%)	Dissipation (%)	Resultant BAC (%)	Comments
7:30 a.m.	0	0	0	0	Entered Bar
8:30 a.m.	3	0.07	0.02	0.05	
9:30 a.m.	3	0.12	0.02	0.10	
10:30 a.m.	3	0.17	0.02	0.15	
11:30 a.m.	3	0.22	0.02	0.20	Last drink
12:30 p.m.	0	0.27	0.02	0.25	
1:30 p.m.	0	0.25	0.02	0.23	Accident
2:04 p.m.	0	0.23	0.01	0.22	Blood draw

Note: Values are rounded to the second decimal place. At each hour, BAC of 0.07 for three drinks consumed is added to the resultant BAC to get the expected BAC.

At a BAC of 0.1%, an experienced chronic alcoholic may appear sober and at a BAC of 0.2%, this individual is expected to show visual signs of intoxication such as loss of coordination, staggering, and slurred speech. However, it is known that chronic alcoholics are often able to mask many of the signs of acute alcohol intoxication, even when there is physiological impairment. Thus, a chronic alcoholic with a BAC of 0.15% to 0.20% may superficially appear sober even when there is impairment of the reflexes, visual acuity, memory, concentration, and judgment **(10)**. The police officer did observe Mr. Bettis and noted in his report that he had only faint alcoholic breath immediately after the accident. His speech was normal but not slurred. His attitude was cooperative. Therefore, it is no wonder that the bartenders serving alcohol could not observe visual effects of alcohol intoxication on Mr. Bettis when he was served his last drink.

17.5.5 Prozac

Prozac is an antidepressant drug and a selective serotonin reuptake inhibitor (SSRI). The liver metabolizes this drug and approximately 95% of this drug is bound to serum proteins. A single oral dose gives peak plasma levels in 6 to 8 hours. The half-life of this drug is approximately 1 to 3 days after a single dose and 4 to 6 days after chronic administration (**13-15**). This drug is prescribed for depression. This drug interferes with cognitive and motor functions and may impair judgment, thinking, and motor skills. Patients are advised to avoid driving a car and are advised not to drink alcohol while on this drug (**13-15**). When a pharmacy fills a prescription for Prozac, this warning is clearly given in writing to the patient. The combined effects of Prozac and alcohol may increase the chance of severity of drowsiness, slowed refluxes, and impaired judgment (**13-15**). This accident was waiting to happen due to Prozac and alcohol in the system of Mr. Bettis. It may be argued that Mr. Bettis takes Prozac every day and an accident had not happened before. However, Mr. Bettis takes Prozac in the morning before he goes to work, but apparently does not drink. However, on the day of the accident he took Prozac before he entered the bar and then consumed several alcoholic drinks. Therefore, this accident happened due to the combined effects of Prozac and alcohol.

17.5.6   Conclusions

It can be concluded with a reasonable degree of scientific and medical certainty that:

1. Mr. Bettis is an alcohol abuser and a chronic alcoholic.
2. This experienced chronic alcoholic did not show visual signs of intoxication to the bartenders or to the police.
3. Mr. Bettis is negligent and irresponsible in drinking alcohol and operating a motor vehicle while on Prozac.
4. This accident was caused by the synergistic effects of Prozac and alcohol.
5. The bartender could not have observed the visual signs of intoxication of Mr. Bettis.

17.6   Alcohol, Multiple Car Crashes, and Traumas

17.6.1   Legal Aspects: Intoxicated Driver, Multiple Car Crashes, and Injuries

This case is another example of a bar violating its responsibility in serving alcoholic beverages to a visually intoxicated person. This resulted in multiple car crashes. Drivers were extricated from their cars. There were several injuries and traumas. One female victim, Melisa, suffered permanent health consequences. Melisa is suing the bar for its negligence in serving alcoholic beverages to an intoxicated driver, which caused the accident and resulted in her pain, suffering, and economic loss.

17.6.2 Medical Aspects: Intoxication of Alcohol

Correlation of blood alcohol levels, the alcohol levels that reach the brain, and the intoxicating effects they produce are well understood. Alcohol intoxication severely impairs driving skills.

17.6.3 Factual Background

An accident involving multiple cars on November 21, 2003 resulted in serious traumas. According to police, the crash occurred at 7:02 p.m. This accident was a consequence of DUI by one of the drivers, Mr. Jerry Reddy. Jerry is a Caucasian male, 28 years of age, 6 feet 2 inches tall and weighing 160 pounds on the day of the accident.

When the police arrived at scene, the Fire Department of Bellow Grove Township was tending to Jerry and two other victims involved in the crash. Jerry was trapped inside his vehicle and had to be extricated from his green Ford Taurus two-door sedan. Deputy Rose Bensen, who was at the scene, observed that the defendant sustained multiple traumas. The defendant and Melisa Getsenbaum, whose car was hit head-on by Jerry's car, were transported by ambulance to St. Mary's Health System. Another victim was sent to University of Xyport Emergency Room.

Jerry's car was eastbound on Curry Road. Melisa's car was westbound. Jerry's car suddenly crossed the lane and hit Melisa's car head-on. Jerry's car then spun around and came to rest in a ditch on the north side of the road. After Melisa's car was hit by Jerry's car, the vehicle spun around and collided with another car that was traveling westbound. Melisa's car came to rest in the westbound lane facing east. One of the cars clipped another vehicle, which was traveling behind the defendant's car.

After finishing the preliminary investigation at the scene, Deputy Rose Bensen made contact with Jerry at St. Mary's Hospital trauma room. She noticed a strong odor of intoxicants from Jerry. He admitted drinking beer at Surya's Bar. He estimates that his last drink was 20 minutes before he left the bar. The hospital determined Jerry's BAC to be 0.207% in a sample of blood drawn at 8:03 p.m. on November 21, 2003.

17.6.4 Medical Consequences of Defendant's DUI

Besides damage to several automobiles involved in the crash and economic consequences suffered by Melisa, Jerry, and several other victims, the accident also resulted in serious medical consequences because of Jerry's severe alcohol intoxication and DUI. Jerry sustained a shattered left arm and had a plate put in with nine screws. He had six broken ribs, punctured lungs, a lacerated spleen, and a broken finger. The nerve damage to his left arm was permanent. Melisa was terrified by the accident. She had excruciating pain, had difficulty breathing, and could not move her leg. She was in the hospital for 40 days. She had severe whiplash, her sternum was fractured, and she had three broken ribs. Her hip was fractured. Her leg was shattered. She had compound fractures of her ankle. She developed infection around her lungs. Even after many days, her ankle was still swollen. Her hip does not have full range of motion. Another victim, Scott Briks, had an injury to his right leg.

17.6.5 Blood Alcohol Concentration

BAC depends upon the time lapse between the last drink and the time of blood draw for alcohol measurement. For a normal healthy man weighing 200 pounds, one alcoholic drink gives a BAC of 0.02%. In the same individual, alcohol is dissipated at a rate of 0.02% in 1 hour (6-10). The defendant weighed 160 pounds; therefore, one alcoholic drink is expected to give a BAC of 0.025%.

Surya's Bar is very close to Jerry's workplace. He worked from 7:00 a.m. to 4:00 p.m. He went to Surya's between 4:00 p.m. to 4:15 p.m. Soon he started drinking beer and probably shots of liquor as well. Jerry admitted that he had previous DUI convictions, that he drinks a 6-pack of beer every day, and he has been drinking for the past 2 years. He admitted that he was intoxicated at the bar and left the bar at approximately 6:30 p.m. He also admitted that he was loud and probably shouting foul language, slurred his words, and was staggering. He says that his last drink was approximately 20 minutes before he left the bar, which may be around 6:00 p.m. or 6:10 p.m. He had no dinner except a few snacks that were on the table. He drank 12-oz. bottles of beer and shots of hard liquor. He does not remember exactly how many he had. His co-workers did not remember how many drinks Jerry had that evening. Jerry admits that he was fuzzy at the bar and he does not remember anything that took place. Was it possible that he was visibly intoxicated at the bar? He admits that it was likely.

Based on this information as well as the BAC determined at the hospital laboratory, it is possible to calculate the defendant's BAC at various times.

Time (h)	Expected BAC (%)	Comments
4:00 p.m.	0	
5:00 p.m.	0.12	
6:00 p.m.	0.24	Last drink
6:30 p.m.	0.23	Left bar
7:00 p.m.	0.22	Accident
8:00 p.m.	0.20	Blood draw

The BAC determined by the hospital was 0.20 at 8:00 p.m. and his last drink was at 6:00 p.m. Between his last drink and the blood draw, the BAC cannot be accumulated but rather dissipated at a rate of 0.02% per hour. Based on this, Jerry's BAC can be calculated easily by adding 0.02% for each hour until his blood draw. The BAC at the time of his last drink would be 0.24%. From the time he entered the bar until he had his last drink, the BAC would be due to accumulation and dissipation. The defendant weighed 160 pounds; therefore, one alcoholic drink gives a BAC of 0.025% and he is expected to dissipate 0.02% alcohol from his blood in 1 hour. When the accident happened, his BAC was calculated to be 0.22% and when he left the bar at 6:30 p.m., the BAC would be 0.23%.

The toxic effects of alcohol intoxication are well documented. Between 0.07% and 0.1% BAC, alcohol intoxication results in impairment of reaction responses, visual acuity, sensory motor coordination, and judgment. Between 0.1% and 0.2% BAC, all of the previously mentioned effects occur and there is a progressive increase in drowsiness, disorientation, and emotional ability. At and above 0.2% BAC, a person is expected to be staggering, grossly impaired, drunk, lethargic, sleepy, or hostile and may pass out. Sometimes a chronic alcoholic may appear sober at 0.1% BAC and yet he will still have the intoxicating effects of alcohol. A chronic alcoholic is expected to exhibit visual effects of alcohol intoxication such as slurring, staggering, and sleepiness, and may pass out at 0.2% BAC (10). By his own admission, Jerry exhibited all of these effects at the bar. The bartender or the waiter could not have missed Jerry's visual effects of alcohol intoxication and yet he was served alcoholic beverages until 20 minutes before he left the bar at 6:30 p.m. The crash resulted in serious traumas at 7:02 p.m. and was definitely due to the alcohol intoxication of Jerry, a consequence of alcoholic beverages served to him at the bar.

17.6.6 Conclusions

It can be concluded with a reasonable degree of scientific and medical certainty that:

1. Jerry Reddy was intoxicated with a BAC of at least 0.22% at the time of the crash.
2. Jerry's BAC remained above 0.2% for at least one hour before he left the bar. He definitely exhibited the visible effects of alcohol intoxication by his own statements.
3. The bar was negligent and irresponsible in serving the defendant alcoholic beverages even after he exhibited visible symptoms of alcoholic intoxication.

4. The irresponsible actions of Surya's Bar and Jerry resulted in multiple car crashes, serious traumas, serious health consequences, suffering, and economic loss to Melisa.

17.7   Intoxicated Passenger Jumps off Wife's Car

17.7.1   Legal Aspects: Intoxicated Passenger Jumps off a Moving Vehicle

This case is about an accident on July 28, 2001 at approximately 9:45 p.m. For unknown reasons, Scott Mullen jumped out of the Land Rover his wife was driving. He received multiple lacerations and injuries and fractured his right ankle. Diana Mullen, his wife, brought a civil lawsuit against the bar for serving alcohol to her husband when he was intoxicated, which caused him to jump out of the Land Rover and sustain multiple injuries. She demands monetary compensation for her husband's pain and suffering.

17.7.2   Medical Aspects: BAC and Intoxication Alcohol

The pharmacokinetics of alcohol are well established. The level of alcohol reaching the brain depends on BAC, which in turn would correlate well with intoxicating effects of alcohol.

17.7.3   Factual Background

Scott Mullen, a Caucasian male, 39 years of age, weighed 165 pounds on the day of the accident, July 28, 2001. He did not complete high school but got his GED. He worked as a carpet installer. He and his wife, Diana Mullen, 36 years of age, were married for 15 years. Diana also did not graduate from high school but got her GED. She worked for a trucking company. According to her testimony, Scott drank between 1 and 20 beers and occasionally a shot of whiskey every day. She also drinks occasionally with her husband. She stated that her husband was previously charged with DUI, spent time in jail, and attended Accelerated Rehabilitative Disposition (ARD) classes. According to her, when her husband gets intoxicated, he exhibits a sluggish walk and his left eye would close. She and Scott's mother were concerned and cautioned him about his excessive drinking. According to Scott, sometimes he would have a couple of roadies, a term used to denote drinking while driving.

On July 28, 2001, Scott and Diana decided to celebrate their 15th wedding anniversary. Scott came home from work and had a couple of beers before they left the house to go to Diana's parents' house where they expected to have a party with other friends and relatives. They put a case of beer in their Jeep before going to Diana's parents' house. Scott says that he probably had a couple of roadies. They arrived at Diana's parents' house at approximately 6:00 p.m. Relatives and friends were there and they obviously had good time. According to Avee Homes, Diana's sister, Scott was drinking heavily. He pinched her at the party. Denzel Ray, who was dating Diana's sister, was also at the party. He says he knew that Scott drank a lot of alcohol.

After two hours at the party, Diana and Scott left. She drove their Land Rover and arrived at Friendly Chaps Inn at approximately 8:00 p.m. Scott ordered one 12-oz. Coors Light beer, which he consumed right away, and Diana ordered a beer and dinner for both of them. Scott got another beer. Before the dinner arrived, Scott ordered a double shot of Firewater. He did not eat dinner but drank approximately half of Diana's beer as well. In all, he consumed at least 2 1/2 beers and one double shot of Firewater. Diana says that her husband once tripped over a bar stool while going to the restroom, which was approximately 15 feet away. According to the testimony of the bartender, Jeremy Strong, he did not notice any visible signs of intoxication in Scott. The couple left the bar and went to the parking lot. They both got into the Land Rover and Scott put on his seat belt. Diana was driving the Land Rover. According to her, they got into an argument and Scott wanted to get out of the car. Diana refused to stop the vehicle because they were close to their house. Scott unbuckled his seat belt and jumped out of the vehicle when it was moving at approximately 35 mph.

According to the Chatville Community Ambulance trip report, the ambulance arrived at the 500 block of Wedge Road at approximately 9:54 p.m. Scott was injured with visible lacerations but was alert and oriented. He was taken to Chatville Medical Center Emergency Room. Scott had injuries and possibly fractured his right ankle. The hospital emergency room doctors also found him to be alert and oriented. His blood was drawn at 10:59 p.m. His BAC was 0.25%. He told the physicians that he jumped out of the moving Land Rover because of his stupidity. While the treatment was in progress, he left the hospital without being discharged. The hospital dispatched police and an ambulance to get him back as he had a fractured ankle. Instead, his wife decided to drive him back herself in her Land Rover to avoid the cost of an ambulance. Scott said that he left the hospital without completing treatment because he was angry. After he came back to the hospital, his treatment was completed and he was subsequently discharged.

17.7.4 Blood Alcohol Concentration

As stated before, BAC depends upon several factors. For a normal healthy male weighing 200 pounds, one alcoholic drink gives a BAC of 0.02%. The same individual dissipates 0.02% alcohol from blood in 1 hour (7,10-12).

17.7.5   Calculation of BAC

It is not known how many drinks Scott Mullen consumed before he entered the Friendly Chaps Inn. However, the number and the type of drinks served at Friendly Chaps Inn are known. His BAC determined at Chatville Hospital is known. Based on this evidence, it is possible to calculate his BAC when the bar started serving drinks at 8:05 p.m. It is scientifically accepted that a 150-pound man will have a BAC of 0.025% after drinking 1 oz. of 50% alcohol (13).

$$BAC = 150 \div \text{Body weight} \times \text{\% ethanol content} \div 50 \times \text{ounces consumed} \times 0.025$$

Coors Light beer has 4.2% alcohol (14) and Firewater has 50% alcohol.

BAC contributed by a total of 30 oz. of Coors Light beer (two beers Scott ordered plus half of Diana's beer):

$$= 150 \div 165 \times 4.2 \div 50 \times 30 \times 0.025 = 0.057\%$$

Rounding to the second decimal place, it would be 0.06%.

BAC contributed by one double shot of Firewater:

$$= 150 \div 165 \times 50 \div 50 \times 2 \times 0.025 = 0.045\%$$

Rounding to the second decimal place, it would be 0.05%.

Total BAC contributed by the drinks served to Scott at Friendly Chaps Inn is

$$0.06 + 0.05 = 0.11\%$$

To find out Scott's BAC just before he entered the bar and was served drinks at the Friendly Chaps Inn, one has to deduct 0.11% (the BAC contributed by drinks served at Friendly Chaps Inn) from 0.25%, the BAC determined at the hospital.

The following table illustrates his calculated BAC at the time his drinks were served at the Friendly Chaps Inn. This table should be read from bottom to top.

Time (h)	BAC (%)	Dissipation (%)	Calculated BAC (%)	Comments
8:00 p.m.		0.06	0.20	Drinks served
9:00 p.m.		0.04	0.18	
9:30 p.m.		0.03	0.17	
10:00 p.m.		0.02	0.16	
10:30 p.m.		0.01	0.15	
11:00 p.m	0.25–0.11	0.14	0	0.14—Blood draw

Alcohol is expected to be absorbed completely in approximately 30 minutes.

Alcohol is dissipated from blood at a rate of 0.02% per hour.

Based on these calculations, Scott's BAC was 0.20% when his drinks were served at Friendly Chaps Inn at 8:05 p.m. His BAC determined at the hospital was 0.25%.

17.7.6   BAC and Signs/Symptoms of Intoxication

Alcohol is a water-soluble compound, and reaches peak blood levels once it is absorbed from the GI tract and then distributed into body compartments. The pharmacology of alcohol and its toxic kinetics are well known. There is a perfect correlation between the BAC and the alcohol levels reaching the brain, and their effect on the CNS and impairment of physiological functions. At a BAC of 0.1% to 0.2%, inexperienced drinkers show visual signs of intoxication such as drowsiness, slurred speech, staggering, gross impairment, and disorientation (7,10).

However, chronic alcoholics develop tolerance to ethanol and are often able to conceal the more overt signs and symptoms of intoxication (10). Most deaths occur at a BAC of 0.4% or higher in inexperienced drinkers. Chronic alcoholics have been apprehended operating motor vehicles with a BAC of 0.4% to 0.5% and have actually survived BACs of 0.6% to 0.7% (7,10).

17.7.7   Alcohol Intoxication of Scott Mullen

Based on the testimony of his wife, relatives, and friends, Scott Mullen is capable of handling large quantities of alcohol. He drinks between 1 to 20 beers every day and has an occasional shot of hard liquor. He was a chronic alcohol abuser for many years. He acquired a tolerance to alcohol.

His tolerance to alcohol is also confirmed by the testimony of others who knew Scott. They say that Scott drank all day and did not exhibit visible signs and symptoms of alcohol intoxication.

There is no evidence that the bartender observed any classical visible signs and symptoms of Scott's alcohol intoxication. The restroom is only about 15 feet from the bar and Scott went to the restroom only once before the drinks were served. There is no evidence that the bartender observed any sluggish walk by Scott. His wife says his left eye was sluggish and closed. This is not a classical symptom of alcohol intoxication.

Diana says her husband was intoxicated when the double shot of Firewater was served before the meal. She could have prevented her husband from buying the double shot of Firewater. There is no evidence that the bartender recognized any manifestations of alcohol intoxication of

Scott. If he did, he probably would not have served the double shot of Firewater.

The paramedics who arrived at the scene of the accident and the hospital personnel at the emergency room found Scott to be oriented and aware of his actions and surroundings. No speech abnormalities or unusual behaviors were noted. His BAC at these times was 0.27% and 0.25%, respectively. On the other hand, his calculated BAC at the bar when his drinks were served was much lower (0.20%). There is no reason to believe that the bartender observed any visual signs of intoxication at a much lower BAC.

Scott was aware of his surroundings and was aware of the consequences of his actions. He was capable of making a conscious decision to get into the Land Rover his wife was driving, buckle the seat belt, later unbuckle the seat belt, and jump from the moving vehicle.

Pinching his sister-in-law at the party, jumping out of a moving vehicle, and leaving the hospital before treatment for his fractured ankle underscores the fact that Scott sometimes exhibits inappropriate and impulsive behavior. This has nothing to do with alcohol intoxication.

17.7.8 Conclusions

Based on the available evidence, it can be concluded with a reasonable degree of scientific certainty that:

1. Scott Mullen is a chronic alcoholic and developed tolerance to alcohol. He was able to conceal overt visible signs and symptoms of alcohol intoxication.
2. Scott Mullen was served drinks at the Friendly Chaps Inn for only a short period. There is no evidence that the bartender observed any unusual behavior or classical signs of intoxication on the part of Scott Mullen.
3. Diana Mullen must bear some responsibility in not preventing her husband from consuming drinks when she knew he was intoxicated.
4. Scott Mullen was aware of the consequences of his actions. He is solely responsible for the injuries sustained by his jumping out of a moving vehicle.

References

1. Stegmaler, C. Info on bars' legal responsibilities in serving alcohol. *Myrtle Beach Restaurant News*. July 30, 2010.
2. Murphy, E. Blame it on the bars. http://www.cfif.org/htdocs/freedomline/current/guest_commentary/dram_shop_liability.htm.
3. Wikipedia. Dram shop. http://en.Wikipedia.org/wiki/Dram _shop.

4. Schlitt, C.L. Alcohol and bad decisions by individuals and bar owners. http:// nylawthoughts.com/2010/05/07/alcohol-and-bad-decisions-by-individuals -and-bar-owners/.
5. Personal Injury. Dram shop liability. http://www.personal-injury-info.net/ dram-shop-liability.htm.
6. Williams, R.H. and Leikin, J.B. Medico legal issues and specimen collection for ethanol testing. *Lab. Med.* **30**:530–537, 1999.
7. Stowell, A.R. and Stowell, L.I. Estimation of blood alcohol concentrations after social drinking. *J. Forensic Sci.* **43**:14–21, 1998.
8. Lands, W.E.M. A review of alcohol clearance in humans. *Alcohol.* **15**:147–160, 1998.
9. Charlebois, R.C., Corbett, M.R., and Wigmore, J.G. Comparison of ethanol concentrations in blood, serum and blood cells for forensic application. *J. Anal. Toxicol.* **20**:171–178, 1996.
10. Di Maio, D.J. and Di Maio, V.J.M. *Forensic Pathology*, CRC Press, Boca Raton, FL, 1993, 447–450.
11. Snyder, R. and Andrews, L.S. Toxic effects of solvents and vapors. In: *Caserett and Dull's Toxicology: The Basic Science of Poisons.* Klaassen, C.D. (Ed.). McGraw-Hill, New York, 1996, 751–752.
12. Burtis, C.A. and Ashwood, E.R. *Tietz Textbook of Clinical Chemistry*, 2nd ed. W.B. Saunders Company, Philadelphia, PA, 1994, 1171.
13. Karch, S.B. *Karch's Pathology of Drug Abuse*, 3rd ed. CRC Press, Boca Raton, FL, 2001.
14. Coors Light. www.summerstage.org/sponsors/coorslight.htm.

Test for Recent Alcohol Use

18

In this chapter, a case illustrates the urine alcohol test to detect the scent of alcohol. Such tests, if available, would be quite useful for law enforcement as well as for medical management. Patients with end-stage liver disease come for liver transplants. Doctors would like to wean such patients from alcohol. To make sure that they abstain from alcohol before they put in a new liver, they are tested for the presence of alcohol in their blood. Law enforcement would like to have a test to detect recent alcohol use. Thus far, no such reliable test is available.

18.1 Urine Test for Recent Alcohol Use (2006–2007)

18.1.1 Legal Aspects: Urine Test for Recent Alcohol Use

This case is about Beverly Binghamton, who is a registered nurse. While working at a nursing home she became addicted to pain medications. She obtained these by misrepresentation. She was apprehended, which resulted in the suspension of her license. She agreed to random urine tests for drugs and alcohol as a part of a deal to restore her license. She continues to be negative for controlled substances in her random urine tests. Her random urine was tested for EtG as a marker for recent alcohol use and these tests were sometimes positive and sometimes inconclusive. She contends that she is not drinking alcohol and challenges the accuracy of the urine test.

18.1.2 Medical Aspects: EtG in Urine Presumptively Indicates Recent Alcohol Use

The principle is because a small amount of unconverted ethanol reacts with UDP-glucuromyl transferase forming ethylglucuronide (EtG), which is excreted in the urine even in the absence of ethanol in the serum. In order to rule out accidental or unintentional exposure to alcohol by foods and hygienic products, a cutoff value of 500 ng/ml was established. This test is now being used to ascertain compliance by healthcare professionals who are being monitored for alcohol use by random urine test for EtG.

18.1.3 Factual Background

Beverly Binghamton is a registered nurse. She is married, lives with her husband, and has no children. Her past medical history includes hepatitis B and hepatitis C. She has chronic hepatitis C infection. She is not diabetic to date. Beverly works during the day at Silvery Nursing Home. Beverly became addicted to prescription pain medications and she obtained them by misrepresentation. She was apprehended in 1999 and prosecuted in 2000. She pled guilty and received three years of probation from the court. The state licensing board suspended her license for 5 years. In 1999, Beverly was an inpatient at the Caron Foundation for treatment of her addiction, followed by outpatient meetings, which lasted many months. She had to wait until her charges were resolved before the Board would accept her into the Professional Health Monitoring Programs (PHMP). During this interim, she independently obtained regular urine screens and had written confirmation of her attendance at all relapse prevention meetings. Furthermore, she also continued with her 12-step meetings, which were presented to the Board prior to her acceptance into the PHMP in January 2001. PHMP involves random urine tests for controlled substances including alcohol. She continues to be negative for controlled substances in her random urine tests.

The Department of Health, State of Ohio sends the random urine samples to Ip Toxicology Laboratory. They measure EtG in urine as a biomarker of recent alcohol use.

18.1.4 EtG as a Marker for Recent Alcohol Use

Testing for recent alcohol use is necessary to monitor compliance of patients when they are being weaned from chronic alcohol use when they come for a liver transplant.

Physicians make sure that these patients are free from alcohol use before they transplant the donor liver. Gama glutamyltranspeptidase (GGT) and carbohydrate deficient transferin (CDT) are used as biomarkers in serum to detect recent alcohol use but with limited success (1). It was established that a major portion of alcohol is metabolized in the liver by ADH, yet a small dose of ethanol (0.02%) is conjugated by UDP-glucuronyl transferases to form EtG and this is excreted in the urine. When unchanged ethanol and metabolites are excreted up to 24 hours, EtG continues to be excreted up to 80 hours in the urine. Thus, even in the absence of ethanol in the urine, the presence of EtG indicates alcohol use (1-6). Analytical methods became available to quantitate EtG by immunoassays and confirmations are done by LC-MS. In order to rule out accidental or unintentional exposure to alcohol by food and hygienic products, a cutoff value of 500 ng/ml was established. This test is now being used to identify compliance of abstaining from alcohol use by healthcare professionals. This is done by monitoring random urine test for EtG (1-6). The presence of EtG in urine is an indication that a person is not abstaining from alcohol use. Problems begin to appear about the specificity of these EtG tests. Several nurses and other health care professionals including pharmacists and doctors protested that even when they are not drinking alcohol intentionally, they are positive for EtG in random urine samples.

18.1.5 Random Urine Tests of Beverly Binghamton

In 2005, Beverly tested positive for alcohol. The state extended her term of random urine testing for another three years. She tested positive for urine alcohol in August 2006, and when contested the state retested her urine sample for alcohol and found the test was negative. In December 2006, the random urine test gave a positive ethanol and retesting also produced a positive ethanol. LC-MS analysis on January 31, 2008 gave an EtG level of 726 ng/ml with a cutoff of 500 ng/ml. On June 14, 2008, Beverly was tested for urine alcohol and found to be positive. She was retested on June 16, 2008 and the result of this test was not communicated to her. She feels that she was probably negative for alcohol at this testing. Thus, her urine alcohol testing by the state gave inconsistent results. Beverly contends that she is not drinking alcohol and wonders how her urine could be testing positive. She says that she is exposed to hygienic products containing substantial levels of alcohol. She probably inadvertently consumed foods or indirectly ingested products that contained alcohol. She feels that there may be problems in the random urine alcohol testing by the state. The urine samples are sent to Ip Toxicology Laboratory. The laboratory offers testing for the presence of EtG in urine as a biomarker for recent alcohol use. Evidence is accumulating that the specificity of this test could be challenged. The medical review officer for the laboratory is Geeta Nathan, MD who is knowledgeable in interpreting the results of controlled substances and alcohol in urine and correlating them with the clinical condition of the person whose urine is being tested.

18.1.6 False-Positive Urine EtG of Beverly Binghamton

It is true that Beverly was apprehended for obtaining prescription pain medications and was prosecuted. She pled guilty and was placed on three-year's probation. Her license was suspended for 5 years. She was subjected to random urine testing for controlled substances. Indeed, she never tested positive for controlled substances during these random urine tests. Alcohol was never an issue and yet she was subjected to random EtG testing. She was surprised that she tested positive in some random urine tests even though she did not intentionally ingest alcohol. She contends that she was probably exposed to products containing alcohol during patient care in the nursing home where she works. She also used mouthwash that contains a substantial amount of alcohol. She presented evidence that when she had an ulcer on her tongue, her dentist asked her to use a mouthwash containing a high amount of alcohol. She has been in communication with other individuals such as nurses and other healthcare professionals including pharmacists and doctors across the country via the Internet. These individuals also encountered positive EtG tests despite abstaining from alcohol use. Beverly had hepatitis B and she now has chronic hepatitis C. She contends that her hepatitis infection probably has something to do with her being EtG positive despite abstaining from alcohol use. She presented supporting letters from her supervisors at work who vouch for her professionalism and honesty. In addition, there is no evidence of alcohol abuse. All of this evidence was presented to the Medical Review Officer who refuses to consider the evidence that she does not abuse alcohol, and insists on taking the EtG results at face value.

18.1.7 Questionable Accuracy of EtG Testing in Random Urine

Even though the presence of EtG is supposed to indicate recent alcohol use, the specificity and sensitivity of this test in various situations is not validated.

- This test was not validated with enough controls that never drank alcohol (4).
- The EtG production in humans varies due to variation in genetic polymorphism in UDP-glucuronyltransferase, the enzyme system that generates EtG from alcohol. Thus, different individuals generate different EtG with the same amount of alcohol ingested (4).
- How body weight, gender, and environmental exposure to ethanol such as medications and hygienic products by inhalation as well as use of hormonal substances affect EtG production is not tested (4).
- One of the serious flaws in EtG testing is the role of endogenous ethanol. There are several cases reported in the literature that confirm that a high carbohydrate diet in the presence of active GI tract fungal infections generates endogenous ethanol causing such patients to become intoxicated with alcohol (7-11). Such endogenously produced ethanol could be converted to EtG (4). Indeed UDP–glucuronyltransferases are expressed in hepatic and extra-hepatic tissues such as colon, kidney, and tissues generating steroids (12-14).
- Ethanol is metabolized mainly in the liver to acetaldehyde and then to acetate. However, a developmental delay in the expression of ADH results in high blood alcohol levels (15). This alcohol could easily be converted to EtG. Such cases of high blood alcohol levels are documented in the scientific literature (15, 16).

- In one case where a patient drank only non-alcoholic beer, his serum alcohol levels were high because he could not metabolize even the very little amount of alcohol present in non-alcoholic beer. The patient had liver cirrhosis and had very little functional liver resulting in high blood alcohol (**17**).
- Hepatitis B and hepatitis C infections result in liver necrosis. The patient may function even with the presence of very little leftover functional liver (**18,19**). Under such circumstances, these patients could not metabolize whatever little ethanol they were inadvertently exposed to through food and hygienic products containing ethanol. Thus, this ethanol may give a positive EtG.
- EtG testing in urine is not currently approved by the FDA and is not used to monitor federal employees.

18.1.8   Conclusions

Based on medical and scientific literature, it can be concluded with a reasonable degree of scientific certainty that Beverly Binghamton:

1. Has liver necrosis due to hepatitis resulting in deficiency of functional liver and ADH.
2. Is exposed to hygienic and cleaning products containing significant alcohol content both at her workplace and in her home. These products are contributing to her endogenous ethanol.
3. Has a presence of extra hepatic UDP-glucuronyl transferases that converts her endogenous ethanol to EtG, which is excreted in her random urine samples.
4. Is not abusing drugs or ethanol.

References

1. Laposta, M. Assessment of ethanol intake–current tests and new assays on the horizon. *Am. J. Clin. Pathol.* **112**:443–450, 1999.
2. Skipper, G.F., Weinmann, W., Thierauf, A., Schaefer, P., Wiesbeck, G., Allen, J.P., Miller, P., and Wurst, F.M. Ethyl glucuronide: Biomarker to identify alcohol use by health professionals recovering from substance use disorders. *Alcohol & Alcoholism*, **39**:445–449, 2004.
3. Wurst, F.M., Vogel, R., Jachar, K., Varga, A., Alling, C., Alt, A., and Skipper, G.E. Ethylglucuronide discloses recent covert alcohol use not detected by standard testing in forensic psychiatric inpatients. *Alcoholism* **27**:471–476.
4. Ethylglucuronide. What is ethylglucuronide? http://ethylglucuronide.net.

5. Dahal, H., Stephanson, N., Beck, O., and Helander, A. Comparison of urinary excretion characteristics of ethanol and ethylglucuronide. *J. Anal. Toxicol.* **26**:201–204, 2002.

6. Wurst, F.M., Wiesbeck, G.A., Metzger, J.W., Weinman, W., and Graf, M. On sensitivity, specificity, and the influence of various parameters on ethyl glucuronide levels in urine–results from the WHO/ISBRA study. *Alcoholism* **28**:1220–1228, 2004.

7. Ladkin, R.G. and Davis, J.P.N. Rupture of stomach in an African child. *Brit. Med. J.* **1**:644, 1948.

8. Kaji, H., Asanuma, Y., Yahara, O., Shihue, H., Hisamura, M., Saito, N., Kawakami, Y., and Murao, M. Intragastro-intestinal alcohol fermentation syndrome: report of two cases and review of literature. *J. Forensic Sci.* **24**:461–471, 1984.

9. Mezey, E., Imbembo, A.L., Potter, J.J., Rent, K.C., Lombardo, R., and Holt, P.R. Endogenous ethanol production and hepatic disease following jejunoileal bypass for morbid obesity. *Am. J. Clin. Nutr.* **28**:1277–1283, 1975.

10. Danshan, A. and Donovan, K. Auto-brewery syndrome in a child with short gut syndrome: case report and review of literature. *J. Ped. Gastroenterol. Nutr.* **33**:214–215, 2001.

11. Spinucci, G., Guidetti, M., Lanzoni, E., and Pironi, L. Endogenous ethanol production in a patient with chronic intestinal pesudo-obstruction and small intestinal bacterial overgrowth. *Eur. J. Gastroenterol. Hepatol.* **18**:799–802, 2006.

12. Chowdhury, J.R., Novikoff, P.M., and Roy, N. Distribution of UDP-glucuronosyl transferases. *Proc. Natl. Acad. Sci.* **82**:2990–2994, 1985.

13. Fisher, M.B., Paine, M.F., Strelevitz, T.J., and Wrighton, S.A. The role of hepatic and extrahepatic UDP-glucuromosyltransferases in humans. *Drug Metabolism.* **33**:273–297, 2001.

14. Gregory, P.A., Lewinsky, R.H., Gadner-Stephen, D.A., and Mackenzie, P.I. Regulation of UDP-glucuronosyltransferases in the gastrointestinal tract. *Toxicol. Appl. Pharmacol.* **15**:354–363, 2004.

15. Wu, H.B., Kelly, M.C., Ostheimer, D., Forte, E., and Hill, D. Definitive identification of exceptionally high methanol concentration in an intoxication of surviving infant: methanol metabolism by first order elimination kinetics. *J. Forensic Sci.* **40**:315–320, 1995.

16. Chikwava, K., Lower, D.R., Frongiskakis, S.H., Sepulveda, J.L., Virji, M.A., and Rao, K.N. Acute ethanol intoxication in a 7-month-old infant. *Pediatric. Dev. Pathol.* **7**:400–402, 2004.

17. DiMartini, A.F. and Rao, K.N. Elevated blood ethanol caused by "non-alcoholic" beer. *J. Clin. Forensic. Med.* **6**:106–108, 1999.

18. Kumar, V., Abbas, A.K., Fausto, N., and Aster, J. *Robbins & Cotran Pathologic Basis of Disease*, 8th ed. Saunders, Elsevier, Philadelphia, PA, 2010.

19. Nine, J.S., Moraca, M., Virji, M.A., and Rao, K.N. Serum ethanol determination. Comparison of lactate and lactate dehydrogenase interference in three enzymatic assays. *J. Anal. Toxicol.* **19**:192–196, 1995.

Drug Overdose 19

In this chapter, three cases are presented to highlight the consequences of prescription drug overdoses. Drug overdoses were described in detail in earlier chapters. The three cases presented here had fatal consequences. The toxicity of prescription drugs underscores the fact that they are to be taken as instructed by the pharmacist and the doctor. In spite of this, these drugs are used for unintended purposes. Prescription drugs are also abused and sold illegally.

19.1 Wrongful Death

19.1.1 Legal Aspects: Attempted Suicide, Drug Overdose, and Wrongful Death

This case is about Larry Higgins, who confided to his friends that he was depressed and took several pills of prescription medications to end his life. His friend rushed him to the Cactoor Community Hospital and told the admitting doctor that Larry was not drunk but took several prescription pills to end his life. The doctor felt Larry had alcoholic breath and ordered that he be put in an isolation unit for further investigation until the next morning. A nurse assistant found him dead the next morning. Larry's mother is suing the hospital and the doctor for wrongful death.

19.1.2 Medical Aspects: Toxicity of Prescription Medications

The prescription medications the patient was on included Percocet, Prozac, and Klonapin. The deceased was suffering from pancreatitis for which he was taking pain medications. He was also being treated for post-traumatic stress disorder. The coroner concluded that Mr. Higgins died due to toxicity of oxycodone and fluoxetine.

19.1.3 Factual Background

Larry Higgins was 46 years of age, African American male, and a veteran. He weighed 213 pounds and was 6 feet 1 inch tall on the day of his death on February 10, 1999. He was being treated for post-traumatic stress disorder, which he attributed to his service in Vietnam and the Gulf War. Dr. Joseph

Anabi was treating him for this ailment as an outpatient at Cactoor Community Hospital. Mr. Higgins was also suffering from pancreatitis for which he was taking pain medications. His prescription medications included Percocet, Prozac, and Klonapin. His past medical history included alcohol abuse. However, he was sober since 1997 and he willingly attended Alcoholics Anonymous (AA) meetings. The evening before his death, Mr. Higgins attended an AA meeting. To his friends, he appeared to be in a severe depression and was unsteady. He confided to his friends that he took an overdose of his medications to end his life, but later changed his mind and now wanted to live. This prompted one of his friends, Mr. Bill Dastoor, to rush him to the Cactoor Hospital on the night of February 9, 1999. His friend notified the hospital staff that Mr. Higgins was not drunk but took an overdose of his prescription medications. The admission notes showed that he was slightly confused, restless, and unsteady, with slurred speech and suicidal ideations. There was no mention of alcoholic breath or glassy eyes (1). No STAT blood alcohol test or urine comprehensive drug screens were requested. In spite of this, he was pronounced drunk. All labs were deferred until morning, when his sobriety was supposed to improve. He was put in a locked facility without any monitoring of his vital signs or observations by the nursing staff. At approximately 7:15 a.m. on February 10, 1999 he was discovered unresponsive. When attempts to revive him failed, he was pronounced dead at 7:45 a.m.

Mr. Higgins's body was transferred to the Perser County Coroner's Office and Lakshmi Ramakrishnan, MD performed an autopsy on February 12, 1999. Urine, bile, eye fluid, and chest blood were collected in grey top tubes and were sent to the county toxicology laboratory. The analysis of blood showed 0.02 mg% of fluoxetine, 0.084 mg% of norfluoxetine, and 0.036 mg% of oxycodone. At the hospital, the blood collected before his death showed 0.014 mg% of oxycodone. Urine screen by ADx was positive for benzodazepine, opiates, and oxycodone, and confirmatory tests by GC-MS were positive for Diphenhydramine, oxycodone, hydrocodone, and fluoxetine. There was no alcohol in the blood or urine. It is surprising that the blood was not tested for acetaminophen even though the deceased was taking Percocet. The presence of oxycodone should have alerted the toxicologist to look for acetaminophen. The autopsy conducted by Dr. Lakshmi Ramakrishnan was thorough and scientific. She noted that the body of Mr. Higgins was that of a well-developed, well-nourished, African American man. The stomach contained 100 mL of partially digested food without any trace of drug-like residues such as pills or capsules. The autopsy showed no end-stage liver disease. Mr. Higgins had acute pulmonary edema and congestion, and died because of fluoxetine and oxycodone toxicity. Apparently, Mr. Higgins was not intoxicated with alcohol but died of a prescription drug overdose. Such a death was preventable and should not have occurred.

19.1.4 Toxicology Findings

19.1.4.1 Alcohol

Mr. Higgins was at the hospital by 12:05 a.m. and was examined by a physician who committed him to a locked facility by 1:05 a.m. on the presumption that Mr. Higgins was intoxicated due to alcohol. There was no mention of alcoholic breath or glassy eyes in the physician notes or the notes written by the nurse. His vital signs were otherwise normal except for blood pressure, which was on the low side. He had slurred speech and was unsteady. Otherwise, this apparently healthy individual died sometime between 1:05 a.m. and 7:45 a.m., from the time he was put in the locked facility to the time he was discovered unresponsive. Alcohol can kill and it is known that a blood alcohol level of 0.4% or higher may cause coma and death due to respiratory paralysis. For the sake of argument, if it is assumed that he had a blood alcohol level of 0.4 or higher and this high blood alcohol level killed him, then alcohol must be present in blood or urine during autopsy. A normal healthy male weighing 200 pounds is known to dissipate 0.02% of alcohol from blood in 1 hour. To dissipate alcohol levels of 0.4% or higher, it would take at least 20 hours (1,2). However, the toxicology report from the coroner's laboratory did not show alcohol in blood or in urine. Therefore, it can be concluded with a reasonable degree of scientific certainty that Mr. Higgins was not drunk and alcohol did not kill him. The coroner was right in concluding that Mr. Higgins died due to toxicity of oxycodone and fluoxetine (3).

19.1.4.2 Drug Overdose

It is not possible to know the exact amount of the three drugs he took. However, whatever he took killed him. It is possible to come to a reasonable and scientifically valid estimate of his drug overdose based on the available information such as the concentration of the drugs in his blood during autopsy even though there may be some drug redistribution after death. The following formula can be used to arrive at a reasonable estimate of his drug intake. Use the following formula (4):

$$Q = Vd \times Css$$

where Q = the amount of initial drug taken, Vd = volume of distribution, and Css = concentration in blood.

The testimony of his friend who brought him to the hospital and his symptoms before his death are also helpful. Mr. Higgins had Klonapin, Percocet, and Prozac at his disposal. According to the autopsy report, there was 100 mL of partially digested food material without any presence of undissolved or partially dissolved tablets or capsules. Therefore, whatever drugs Mr. Higgins took were apparently absorbed from the GI tract.

19.1.4.3 Klonopin

Klonopin is a benzodiazepine, which is rapidly absorbed after oral administration. It is available in 0.5-mg, 1-mg, or 2-mg tablets. The elimination half-
life from blood is 30 to 40 hours. During autopsy, Mr. Higgins's blood did not
show any benzodiazepine. Therefore, it is reasonable to conclude that he did
not overdose with this drug, as this drug has a long elimination half-life and
its presence would have been detected in the screen if this drug were indeed
in his blood (3).

19.1.4.4 Prozac

Prozac is an antidepressant and the active ingredient is fluoxetine. It is given
at a dose of 20 to 80 mg/day. The drug is well absorbed in the body with an
elimination half-life of 1 to 3 days for fluoxetine and 4 to 6 days for norfluoxetine, its active metabolite. The toxic effects of this drug in overdose situations
include nervousness, nausea, hypertension, anxiety, disorientation, and CNS
depression. Mr. Higgins exhibited these symptoms when he was brought to
the hospital. It is difficult to arrive at an accurate estimate of the amount of
fluoxetine that was taken based on the levels seen in autopsy blood, as fluoxetine is known to redistribute postmortem. However, a reasonably accurate
estimate of this drug is possible. Here the assumption is that he might have
taken this drug at least 18 hours prior to his death. If this was the case, then
the blood levels seen during autopsy should be multiplied by 1.5 to arrive at
peak blood levels. The Vd is 26 L. Mr. Higgins weighed 84 kg. Therefore, the
approximate loading dose, Q, would be:

$$Q = Vd \times Css$$

$$Css = 0.02mg\% \text{ or } 0.2mg/L \text{ or } 0.3 \text{ peak blood levels.}$$

Therefore,

$$Q = 26 \times 84 \times 0.3 = 655.2 \text{ mg}$$

If it is assumed that he was taking 20 to 40 mg/day, then he overdosed by at
least 15 to 20 times that amount (4).

19.1.4.5 Percocet

Percocet tablets are prescribed essentially to alleviate pain. Mr. Higgins was
suffering from pain due to pancreatitis. Therefore, it is not surprising that
he was using Percocet. Percocet contains 5 mg of oxycodone hydrochloride,
325 mg of acetaminophen, and other inactive ingredients. Percocet tablets
are taken every 6 hours as needed. Oxycodone, like morphine, impairs CNS

functions, causes extreme somnolence progressing to stupor or coma, sedation, dizziness, severe respiratory depression, bradycardia, apnea, circulatory
collapse, cardiac arrest, and death. Its elimination half-life is 4 to 6 hours and
volume of distribution is approximately 1.8 L/kg. If it is assumed, as before,
that Mr. Higgins ingested an overdose of Percocet some 18 hours prior to his
death, then the drug had undergone at least three elimination half-lives in his
blood. The levels found at autopsy were 0.036 mg% or 0.36 mg/L and the peak
blood levels were expected to be around 1.08 mg/L.

It is possible to calculate the dose he took using the following formula:

$$Q = Vd \times Css$$
$$= 1.8 \times 84 \times 1.08$$
$$= 163 \text{ mg}$$

It is reasonable to estimate that he might have taken approximately 163
mg of oxycodone or about 30 tablets of Percocet (3). He consumed at least 8
to 10 times the recommended maximum dose.

It is not possible to know when Mr. Higgins took these drugs. The fact
remains that he confided to his friends that he over-medicated himself,
wanted to live, and was having anxiety and restlessness to get out of this
predicament. For this reason, his friend rushed him to the hospital for timely
medical intervention. This was an unnecessary and preventable death of an
otherwise healthy and well-nourished man.

19.1.5   Conclusions

It can be concluded with a reasonable degree of scientific certainty that:

1. Mr. Higgins died due to fluoxetine and oxycodone toxicity.
2. His death was from a drug overdose.
3. This death was unnecessary and preventable.

19.2   Criminal Homicide

19.2.1   Legal Aspects: Criminal Homicide

This case involves Mr. Rambo McVay, who was charged with first-degree
murder of his girlfriend, Ms. Avee Ashley. They both attempted suicide by
taking an excessive overdose of OxyContin. Avee Ashley died but Rambo
McVay survived and was charged with criminal homicide.

19.2.2   Medical Aspects: OxyContin Toxicity

Oxycodone is a semi-synthetic opiate used in the treatment of pain. It is now available as OxyContin, a time-released pill. If the OxyContin pill is crushed and snorted or injected, it produces a quick heroin-like high oftentimes resulting in death.

19.2.3   Factual Background

This case involves Mr. Rambo McVay who is charged with first-degree murder of his girlfriend, Ms. Avee Ashley. Rambo McVay is a Caucasian male, 56 years of age, and weighing 240 pounds. Avee Ashley was a Caucasian female, 53 years of age, and weighing 140 pounds.

The police and the detective in charge of the case interviewed the defendant. The defendant told them that he and Avee decided to commit suicide on the evening of August 26, 2000. The defendant crushed 30 pills of OxyContin and dissolved this in water. They both drank this during the early evening hours of August 26, 2000. In response to a complaint from Avee's son who was looking for his mother, the police entered the defendant's house on August 27, 2000. They found the defendant unresponsive in his house. The female companion was found lying dead on the bed. The paramedics found the defendant responsive only to pain and noticed a powdery substance around his mouth. There was apparently a suicide note on the wall by the defendant. He was brought to the emergency department of Fastiv County Regional Hospital. The defendant was found to be lethargic at the hospital. Results from the hospital laboratory showed that the defendant was positive for opiates. There was no alcohol or other drugs in the defendant's system.

The defendant previously worked as an ambulance driver and then later as a truck driver. He is at present on Workers' Compensation after a rib injury sustained while driving a truck. Past medical history is remarkable for coronary artery disease, hypertension, non-insulin dependent diabetes, obesity, left rib injury, and left rib and back pain. The defendant also suffered from depression and bipolar disorder. He is a high school graduate who was married four times. According to the police detective, the defendant stated that he got on top of Avee and choked her.

19.2.4   Autopsy

Dr. Chu Wu performed the autopsy on Avee's body. He concluded that death was due to asphyxiation attributable to manual strangulation even though he did not present any physical or pathological evidence to support such a conclusion. Manual strangulation compresses internal structures of the neck resulting in occlusion of the blood vessels. In manual strangulation, the face usually appears congested and cyanotic, with petechiae of the conjunctivae and sclera. In most cases, strangulation marks of violence are usually present on the skin of the neck. Typically, abrasions, contusions, and fingernail marks are seen on the skin. Rarely are no marks present. Dissection of the throat usually reveals hemorrhage. Sometimes there may be fractures of the hyoid bone or thyroid cartilage. The incidence of fractures is high if a careful dissection of the neck is conducted (1). In any case, Dr. Wu did not discuss the presence of evidence or lack of it in his report suggestive of manual strangulation. This is important especially when he is concluding that Avee Ashley died of manual strangulation. His autopsy report did not discuss why he concludes that Avee Ashley's death was not caused by oxycodone overdose.

19.2.4.1   OxyContin

Oxycodon is a semi-synthetic opiate used in the treatment of pain. It is now available as OxyContin, a time-released pill. This drug is used in the treatment of pain with an elimination half-life of 2 to 5.5 hours. It is rapidly absorbed and the time-released formulation is designed to release the drug slowly and be effective up to 12 hours. This drug is now abused for its potential to cause euphoria and feelings of relaxation. The OxyContin pill is chewed or the crushed pill is snorted or injected to produce a quick heroin-like high. This often results in fatalities (2,3). The absorption half-life of the immediate release form is only 0.4 hours and the bioavailability is 100%. The therapeutic objective is to achieve plasma steady state levels of 10 ng/mL to 100 ng/mL. Anything over 200 ng/mL is considered toxic (4,5).

The toxic reactions include respiratory depression, somnolence progressing to stupor, hypotension, nausea, vomiting, and CNS effects. This drug may impair mental and physical ability. Drowsiness, sedation, dizziness, nausea, and vomiting may occur. Agitation, anxiety, confusion, nervousness, neuralgia, personality disorder, and tremors have been reported in some patients. The female subjects on average have higher plasma concentrations of OxyContin than male subjects adjusted for body weight. Detection of OxyContin abuse is problematic as it is cleared from the urine so rapidly and the window of detection is under 24 hours. Little is known about the postmortem toxicology and pathology of OxyContin-related deaths (2). No unique pathological findings are recognized. Again, very little is known about the postmortem redistribution of this drug (1). A recent study by Los Angeles County Coroner's Toxicology Laboratory detected oxycodone in 67 postmortem cases. Of these, 36 were found to be due to controlled release tablets. It was found in these postmortem cases that the heart blood contained 0.12 to 46 mg/L and the femoral blood contained 0.10 to 13 mg/L (5).

Cancer patients on OxyContin therapy do develop tolerance and oftentimes require progressively higher doses. Occurrence of cross-tolerance to other opioids is also known (5). Patients on OxyContin develop physical dependence and the withdrawal symptoms of this drug are characterized by restlessness, lacrimation, rhinorrhea, yawning, perspiration, chills, myalgia, and hydriasis. Other symptoms include irritability, anxiety, backache, joint pain, weakness, abdominal cramps, and insomnia (3,5).

19.2.5 Defendant

As stated earlier, the police entered the defendant's apartment on August 27, 2000 at 11:00 a.m. The paramedics found the defendant to be responsive to pain only. When he was brought to the hospital, the urine drug screen done at 12:32 p.m. was found to be positive for opiates. There were no other drugs or alcohol found in his system. OxyContin, once crushed and taken in, is rapidly absorbed and has an elimination half-life of 2 to 5.5 hours. Oxycodone is cleared from the urine rapidly and its detection in the laboratory is problematic after 24 hours. The fact that it could be detected in the defendant's urine at 12:32 p.m. on August 27, 2000 suggests that the intentional overdose probably occurred within the past 24 hours. The defendant survived but Avee Ashley did not, even though both received the acute overdose. This suggests that Rambo McVay weighed more than Avee Ashley did and because of OxyContin therapy, he probably developed tolerance for the drug (6). Avee Ashley was naïve to OxyContin. Based on the observations of the police and paramedics on the condition of the defendant and the presence of the dead girlfriend at 11:15 a.m. on August 27, 2000, it can be concluded that the intentional overdose occurred in the late evening hours of August 26, 2000.

Increased oxycodone plasma concentration causes dose-related adverse reactions such as nausea, vomiting, CNS effects, and respiratory depression. The defendant indeed had shown these classical symptoms of oxycodone toxicity (3,5). When the police and paramedics found him in his home, he was still suffering from oxycodone intoxication and was not aware of his surroundings. When he was brought to the hospital, he was slowly coming out of OxyContin intoxication. At the hospital, he showed agitation, anxiety, nervousness, confusion, neuralgia, and personality disorder—all symptoms of OxyContin intoxication. The police went to the hospital at 9:45 p.m. on August 27, 2000 and interviewed the defendant. The interview was completed by 10:35 p.m. The fact that the hospital detected the presence of opiates in the defendant's urine supports the conclusions of the toxicologist, Dr. Bernie Klingesberg, that the defendant was suffering from acute side effects of opiate overdose and was incapable of causing the death of Avee Ashley. OxyContin overdose has an effect on mental stability and this probably caused both anterograde and retrograde amnesia. Therefore, the memory of the defendant for the events in question would be unreliable. It is also apparent that the defendant overdosed himself with OxyContin approximately 24 hours earlier and therefore might be undergoing opiate withdrawal, which is characterized by several symptoms including restlessness, lacrimation, chills, myalgia, yawning, perspiration, irritability, anxiety, weakness, and insomnia. Therefore, the interview given by the defendant to the police is unreliable.

19.2.6 Decedent

Avee Ashley was naïve to OxyContin, unlike the defendant who was on OxyContin therapy and probably had developed opiate tolerance and withdrawal. Avee died due to the sudden absorption of the toxic amounts of the drug and the resultant toxic reaction. Moreover, Avee had a lower body weight than the defendant. As stated previously, Avee's autopsy showed the presence of oxycodone in the gastric contents suggesting that the drug was not completely absorbed. The blood toxicology showed a level of 0.24 mg/ml, which is in the toxic range. As stated earlier, the immediate release form of OxyContin has an absorption half-life of 0.4 h and 100% of this is bioavailable (3). The sudden influx of a massive quantity of OxyContin in a female naïve to OxyContin is expected to cause toxic reactions, which include respiratory depression, somnolence progressing to stupor, hypotension, nausea, vomiting, and CNS effects. Little is known about the postmortem toxicology and pathology of OxyContin-related deaths. No unique pathological findings are recognized. In a recent study by Los Angeles County Coroner's Toxicology Laboratory, oxycodone was detected in 67 postmortem cases. Of these, 36 were found to be due to controlled-release tablets. It was found in these postmortem cases the heart blood contained 0.12 to 46 mg/L and femoral blood contained 0.10 to 13 mg/L of oxycodone (5,6). Even though very little is known about the postmortem toxicology and redistribution of this drug (2), we can assume that this drug underwent at least two elimination half-lives of 5 hours each before Avee died. This further supports the contention that the OxyContin intake probably occurred in the late evening hours of August 26, 2000. Lack of physical and pathological evidence at autopsy and the corroboration of the presence of opiate overdose in the defendant and the deceased's blood suggest that OxyContin caused the death of Avee Ashley.

19.2.7 Conclusions

Based on the scientific and medical literature, it can be concluded with a reasonable degree of scientific and medical certainty that:

1. The defendant was suffering from acute oxycodone toxicity, super-imposed with his existing psychiatric illness.
2. There is no physical or pathological evidence to suggest that Avee Ashley died of asphyxiation.
3. Avee Ashley died from an acute overdose of OxyContin.

19.3   Drug Abuse, House Fire, and Death

19.3.1   Legal Aspects: Drug Abuse, House Fire, and Death

This case is about Vicki Pascale, who died in an accidental house fire. The firefighters and police urged her to jump approximately 10 feet from the second-floor bathroom window into their waiting hands. Instead, she went back into the burning house and died. John Pascale, Vicki's father, and Robert Baker, Vicki's boyfriend, brought a civil suit against Bill Bufetaria, the owner of the house for his negligence in not repairing the faulty electrical system, which caused the house fire. The defendant contends that he is not responsible for her death as Vicki Pascale was a chronic drug abuser and the toxic effects of drugs impaired her ability to think, and inhibited her cognitive and perceptual abilities.

19.3.2   Medical Aspects: Toxicity of Drugs

Vicki was a chronic drug abuser, and concomitant use of alprazolam potentiated the toxic effects of marijuana, impaired her ability to think, and inhibited her cognitive and perceptual abilities. She went back into a burning house, which eventually killed her.

19.3.3   Factual Background

This case deals with an accidental house fire resulting in the death of Vicki Pascale, a 26-year-old woman. John Pascale, Vicki's father, and Robert Baker, Vicki's boyfriend, lived in the second-floor apartment in the house. This was a 100-year-old building divided into two apartments.

On the morning of February 6, 2005, at 5:35 a.m. a fire broke out, which was determined to be electrical in nature. Both John Pascale and Robert Baker escaped the fire with nonfatal injuries. When the firefighters and police arrived at the scene, flames were intense. Vicki opened the bathroom window and talked to the firefighters and police who were down below at the scene. The flames were intense and the firefighters and police urged her to jump from the window. The window was only 10 feet above the ground. She refused to jump and went back into the burning house. She eventually was overcome by smoke and fumes, collapsed back into the building, and eventually died. Autopsy was performed on Vicki's body. AxT Diagnostics tested the blood and urine for drugs. The results showed that Vicki was positive for cannabinoids and alprazolam. The coroner established the cause of death as carboxyhemoglobin and smoke inhalation. Vicki's autopsy blood had 18 mg/L of alprazolam. The therapeutic range is 0.1 to 0.2 mg/L. She had 6.4 mg/L of 11-nor-9 carboxy THC. According to AxT Diagnostics, 4 to 20 mg/L of this metabolite in blood is known to occur 12 hours after use. The coroner ruled that the main cause of death was due to house fire (accidental).

19.3.4   Drug Abuse in the Household

The household consisted of Vicki Pascale, her father, John Pascale, and her boyfriend, Robert Baker. Robert Baker is a high school graduate who works as an electrician. At the hospital, he admitted using marijuana and he stated that he and Vicki smoked marijuana that evening before the fire, probably at 6:00 p.m. They both went to bed around 2:30 a.m. The hospital did blood as well as urine drug screens. They revealed the presence of cannabinoids and other narcotic medication. Medical records of John Pascale also showed that he reported depression, anxiety disorder, and chronic back pain. He was on Percocet twice a day. Analysis of his blood collected on August 9, 2004 tested positive for benzodiazepines and oxycodone. A letter from Dr. Eric Bartley indicates that urine analysis earlier showed the presence of drugs not reported by him and not prescribed for him. Medical records of Vicki show several injuries and falls. These records, dated as early as 2002, showed a consistent pattern of self-inflicted violence (SIV) usually associated with chronic drug abusers who try to obtain prescription pain medications. The patient was married before and had a miscarriage. She was referred to Globe Community Behavioral Clinic as an outpatient. The major diagnosis was depression and panic disorder. She used marijuana and caffeine pills. Thus, all of the members of the household used several drugs. It is not surprising that the autopsy of Vicki Pascale revealed the presence of alprazolam and marijuana.

19.3.5   Toxic Effects of Alprazolam and Marijuana

Alprazolam, also known as Xanax, is a benzodiazepine and is prescribed for anxiety disorder at 0.2 mg 2 or 3 times a day. Vicki's autopsy revealed alprazolam at 0.78 mg, which was much above the expected therapeutic range (0.02 to 0.1mg/L). Toxic side effects of this drug include dizziness and coordination difficulties. Irritability and hallucinations were also known to occur. Concomitant use of this drug with alcohol and other CNS drugs is prohibited. It is clearly stated that this drug has a potential for abuse. This drug is sold on the black market. The state of relaxation, anxiolysis, and disinhibition induced by this drug is the main reason for its recreational use. This drug is used with marijuana or heroin to potentiate the relaxing effect (3,7–9). Besides alprazolam, Vicki's autopsy revealed a considerable amount of marijuana in the blood. Her boyfriend confirmed in his deposition that both of them smoked marijuana the evening before the fire. Marijuana toxicity includes short-term memory loss, and inability to accomplish tasks requiring multiple mental steps. A high level of marijuana intoxication decreases motor coordination, muscle strength, and steadiness. Lethargy and sedation are reported. There is a non-linear correlation between plasma THC levels and degree of intoxication. The elimination half-life is approximately 72 hours. Laboratory analysis is by immunoassay. In urine, THC metabolites can be detected up to several days. People smoking marijuana report intense relaxation and elevation of mood followed by drowsiness and sedation. The most important effect is altered perception and loss of ability to problem-solve (10-14).

19.3.6   Conclusions

Based on the evidence available, it can be concluded with a reasonable degree of scientific and medical certainty that:

1. Vicki Pascale was a chronic drug abuser and had toxic levels of alprazolam and marijuana in her blood at the time of the fire and at autopsy.
2. She could have easily jumped 10 feet from the bathroom window to the waiting hands of police and firemen below.
3. Alprazolam present in her blood potentiated the toxic effects of marijuana, impaired her ability to think, and inhibited her cognitive and perceptual abilities resulting in her going back into the burning house, which eventually resulted in her death.

References

1. Di Maio, D.J. and Di Maio, V.J.M. *Forensic Pathology*. CRC Press, Boca Raton, FL, 1994, 446–450.
2. Williams, R.H. and Leikin, J.B. Medico-legal issues and specimen collection for ethanol testing. *Lab. Med.* **30**:530–537, 1999.
3. Basset, R.C. and Cravey, R.H. *Disposition of Toxic Drugs and Chemicals in Man.* Chemical Toxicology Institute, Foster City, CA, 1994.
4. Karch, S.B. *Karch's Pathology of Drug Abuse*, 3rd ed. CRC Press, Boca Raton, FL, 2001.

5. Anderson, D.T., Fritz, K.L., and Muto, J.J. OxyContin: the concept of a "ghost pill" and the postmortem tissue distribution of oxycodone in 36 cases. *J. Anal. Toxicol.* **26**:448–459, 2002.

6. Cleary, J. Translating opioid tolerance research. *APS Bull.* **6**:1–10, 1996.

7. Alprazolam. www.mentalhealth.com, 2007.

8. Wikipedia. Alprazolam. http://en.wikipedia.org/wiki/Alprazolam, 2007.

9. Alprazolam. Micromedix healthcare series, 2007.

10. Marijuana. www.Brown.edu/student_services/health_education/alcohol_ tobacco_&other_drugs/marijuana.php.

11. Marijuana. Micromedix healthcare series, 2007.

12. NIDA. Info facts: Marijuana. www.nida.nih.gov, 2007.

13. Drug facts. Marijuana. www.whitehouse.gov/search/site/marijuana.

14. Marijuana. Medical Review Officer Information. Micromedix healthcare series, 2007.

Toxic Torts

20

In this chapter, several interesting cases that come under tort law are presented. Tort law can be defined as a civil wrong that can be redressed by awarding damages. Among the damages the injured party may recover are loss of earning capacity, pain and suffering, and reasonable medical expenses. There are three types of torts: (1) intentional torts, (2) negligent torts, and (3) strict liability torts (**1**). Under this law, if someone suffers a physical, legal, or emotional harm, the injured party may be able to pursue a lawsuit. If this lawsuit is deemed justified, the victim may be awarded compensation as a remedy for his or her suffering (**2**). Chemical injury (or toxic torts) are included in this chapter. Environmental pollution is included in toxic torts (**3**).

20.1   Toxic Christmas Tree

20.1.1   Legal Aspects: Toxic Christmas Tree

This case involves a 40-year-old Caucasian woman who suffered several health problems because of chlorpyrifos poisoning. Angelina was admitted to the hospital for several health problems including malaise, headache, night sweats, a feverish tendency, nausea, vomiting, abdominal cramps, difficulty moving her bowels, difficulty urinating, and muscle pain. These health problems appeared after she put up a Christmas tree bought from Tixy Farms, the biggest supplier of Christmas trees in Ohio. The supplier sprayed the tree with Dursban Pro. Angelina sued Trixy Farms for monetary compensation for her health problems, including her pain and suffering.

20.1.2   Medical Aspects: Chlorpyrifos Toxicity

Dursban Pro contains chlorpyrifos. The chemical name for chlorpyrifos is O,O-diethyl-O- 3,5,6-trichloropyridin-2-ylphosphorothioate. It is used extensively as a pesticide in agriculture, industry, and households. Angelina put the Christmas tree in her house and was pricked several times by the needles of the tree. Exposure to chlorpyrifos can occur orally, through inhalation, or by absorption through the skin. The acute toxicity of this pesticide causes nausea, vomiting, abdominal cramps, diarrhea, headache, giddiness, vertigo, weakness, tightness of the chest, excessive tearing, ocular pain, blurred vision, loss of muscle coordination, and slurred speech.

20.1.3 Factual Account

Angelina was admitted to the hospital for several health problems including malaise, headache, night sweats, a feverish tendency, nausea, vomiting, abdominal cramps, difficulty moving her bowels, difficulty urinating, and muscle pain. She told her physicians that these symptoms appeared after she bought a Christmas tree from Trixy Farms. She put the Christmas tree in her house and was pricked several times by the needles of the tree. The radiological workup revealed abdominal adhesions. She also saw several physicians including a dermatologist for the acute symptoms as well as skin lesions. The skin lesions first started on her arms, and then spread to her legs, feet, and ankles. Examination by a dermatologist revealed partly blanching erythematosus and voracious macules and papules, some with necrotic centers. The areas involved included the distal forearms, buttocks, and the upper and lower legs extending onto the feet. Skin biopsy revealed cutaneous vasculitis with fibrin thrombi inside the small blood vessels. Angelina told the physicians that when she put up the tree initially, the tree fell on her accidentally and after two weeks the clinical symptoms as noted previously flared up. Her urine analysis by GC-MS was positive for chlorpyrifos. The laboratory findings and her clinical symptoms pointed to diagnosis of organophosphorus insecticide toxicity and chlorpyrifos-induced vasculitis. The man who sold the tree to Angelina admitted spraying the tree heavily with Dursban Pro, which confirmed the diagnosis. The clinicians concluded that the probable mechanism of the skin reactions was likely an immune-complex mediated vasculitis with the antigen being the pesticide. Her clinical symptoms disappeared after treatment with Prednisone. Thus, Angelina suffered chlorpyrifos poisoning, which resulted in her acute and delayed clinical symptoms.

20.1.4 Chlorpyrifos Toxicity

Chlorpyrifos is used extensively as a pesticide in agriculture, industry, and households. As with any pesticide, improper use will result in its toxicity. Because of its extensive use, chlorpyrifos is a major source of exposure among Americans and its exposure appears to be increasing with increase in its use. Exposure to chlorpyrifos can occur orally, through inhalation, or by absorption through the skin. Animal studies in the laboratory revealed that this pesticide is rapidly absorbed through the skin in a matter of minutes. The acute toxicity of this pesticide causes nausea, vomiting, abdominal cramps, diarrhea, headache, giddiness, vertigo, weakness, tightness of the chest, excessive tearing, ocular pain, blurring of vision, loss of muscle coordination, and slurring of the speech (**4**). Indeed, Angelina suffered most of these symptoms suggesting chlorpyrifos toxicity. Different people develop different delayed symptoms. Angelina exhibited most of the acute symptoms as well as skin reactions manifesting as vasculitis. This indicated that inhalation and dermal absorption of chlorpyrifos caused clinical symptoms and skin reactions in Angelina. Medical literature indicates that several office workers showed chlorpyrifos toxicity when this insecticide was sprayed around their building. They developed acute symptoms as well as delayed effects suggesting the redistribution of this compound to a second body compartment and subsequent release of an active principle (**5**).

The onset of organophosphorus insecticide induced skin lesions is documented in the scientific literature, even though such cases are rare. A five-year-old girl was exposed to Filtration and developed skin lesions. These were polymorphic lesions in the form of papules, necrotizing vesicles, and ulcerations. The lesions were detected on the trunk, on the face, and on extremities (**6**). Contact dermatitis due to organophosphorus insecticide was examined in 202 patients showing symptoms of toxicity. Twenty-five percent of these cases showed dermatitis. The causal relationship between organophosphate toxicity and skin lesions was confirmed by animal experiments. Experiments with guinea pigs showed that organophosphorus insecticide caused primary irritating skin reactions and dermatitis was seen in several regions of the body (**7**). This is not surprising in view of the fact that organophosphorus insecticides cause allergic reactions and destroy the ultrastructure of the skin (**8,9**).

20.1.5   Diagnosis of Vasculitis

Based on clinical symptoms and skin biopsy, the dermatologist concluded that Angelina's skin lesions were chlorpyrifos-induced vasculitis with necrotic regions. The dermatologist concluded that the pesticide bound to a protein in her body rendering it immunogenic, and she responded by forming antibodies against it. The protein/pesticide complex binds the antibody and forms a circulating immune complex that, depending on size and net surface change, lodges in blood vessel walls at certain sites in the body. Deposition of immune complexes leads to activation of the vascular endothelial cells, thereby provoking release of vasoactive mediators and high levels of tissue plasminogen activators. This activation influences the vaso-permeability, the tissue deposition of additional immune complexes, and infiltration by inflammatory cells, which release tissue-damaging enzymes into the local environment (**10,11**). This contention is supported by the observation that chlorpyrifos causes immunologic abnormalities in humans. The presence of different types of autoantibodies may indicate generalized tissue injury has occurred (**8**).

20.1.6   Conclusions

Based on the evidence available, it can be concluded that:

1. The acute symptoms and vasculitis seen in Angelina were probably caused by chlorpyrifos that was sprayed on the Christmas tree.
2. The clinicians were right in associating this pesticide with Angelina's acute toxic effects and clinical symptoms.

20.2   Exterminator Mistakes and Health Problems

20.2.1   Legal Aspects: Health Problems of Bank Employees

This case involves five women who worked as tellers at the Putnam Bank, Springfield, Illinois. These five employees suffered serious health problems secondary to exposure to Dursban Pro pesticide spray at the bank. These five women (plaintiffs) filed a lawsuit against the extermination company and its business insurance company (defendants) for monetary compensation for their health problems and for their pain and suffering.

20.2.2   Medical Aspects: Pesticide Toxicity

Dursban Pro contains chlorpyrifos and xylene, an organic solvent. Chlorpyrifos is classified as a Class 3 toxin because it can cause irreversible effects that can be life threatening. It is an organophosphorus pesticide that is a white crystal-like solid with a strong odor that does not mix well with water. Therefore, organic solvents are used before it is applied.

20.2.3   Factual Background

The bank engaged the services of Sure Shot Exterminating Company to get rid of a flea infestation on their premises. The extermination company employees usually come to the bank and treat the bank premises with pesticide. The five tellers who worked there had no complaints on previous occasions. However, on August 15, 1997, the extermination company came to the bank in the late afternoon and sprayed Dursban Pro pesticide on the bank premises including the teller area. The manager closed the bank for the day because the customers and the tellers complained of the intense odor, and they were coughing. The windows and doors were opened and the maintenance staff shampooed the carpet, washed the walls, and put on powerful fans. The next morning the tellers came back to work. They complained of burning eyes, severe headaches, coughs, and shortness of breath. They complained that they were severely poisoned. Employees of the extermination company insisted that they used the correct dilution of the concentrated pesticide solution as recommended by the manufacturer. One bank employee, Amanda, required hospitalization for three days. All the employees subsequently developed long-lasting health problems.

Mr. Benzamin Sarvos, president of the Putnam Bank, became concerned about the persistent health problems of his employees after exposure to the Dursban Pro spray. He invited Dr. Patrick Chang of Environ Health Consultants Inc. to measure the pesticide residues in the bank. Dr. Chang's initial visit was five days after the spray and he subsequently visited the bank on two more occasions. Each time, Dr. Chang took surface and air samples and analyzed them by GC-MS for chlorpyrifos and solvent still present in the sprayed areas. Dr. Chang met with two representatives of the extermination company on his initial visit and was told that they assumed that the correct concentration of Dursban Pro was in their applicators when they sprayed the bank. Dursban Pro contains 22.5% chlorpyrifos, 77.5% solvents, and other materials. The Dow Chemical Company recommends a working solution of 0.25% for routine application and 0.5% solution for heavy infestation. Representatives of the exterminating company thought that they used a 0.25% solution at the bank. However, analysis of the pesticide residues at the bank showed that too much Dursban was sprayed. Dr. Chang very rightly concluded that there could not have been a smell after 5 days if the recommended concentration of Dursban had been sprayed. The analytical results showed that mistakes had been made during the application of Dursban Pro. The smell of solvents in the area confirmed that too much Dursban Pro was sprayed at the bank. The wallpaper also contained chlorpyrifos residue even after 5 months.

20.2.3.1 Employee 1

Diana is a 43-year-old Caucasian female. She had a prior history of mild asthma but was not on any regular medication. She neither smokes nor drinks alcohol. However, after this incident her severe health problems forced her to seek treatment from a primary physician, a pulmonary specialist, and a neurologist. She developed neurological symptoms, loss of sleep, breathing difficulties, carpal tunnel syndrome, sore throat, tightness of chest, nausea, wheezing, and sleep apnea. The diagnosis included small airways dysfunction and bronchial asthma. She was unresponsive to bronchodilators. Thus, the pesticide exposure resulted in permanent health problems for Diana.

20.2.3.2 Employee 2

Brenda is a Caucasian female who was also exposed to the insecticide. However, she had no health insurance and consequently had very little treatment. She waited five days to seek medical treatment. She had burning in her lungs, cough, and felt bad overall. The physician's examination revealed lower lobe pneumonia.

20.2.3.3 Employee 3

Jennifer is a 32-year-old Caucasian woman who had some minor sinus problems before exposure to the insecticide at the bank. Her condition became worse after the exposure and required treatment by a primary physician, an allergist, and a pulmonary specialist. Immediately after the exposure to Dursban, she developed congestion in the head, hoarseness, headache, shortness of breath, burning and swelling of the eyes, and heartburn. The diagnosis included allergic rhinitis.

20.2.3.4 Employee 4

Mary Alan is a 42-year-old Caucasian female with no previous history of asthma, allergies, or hay fever. Immediately after exposure to Dursban Pro at the bank, she developed shortness of breath, wheezing, a burning sensation in her mouth and throat, hoarseness, and headaches. Her symptoms were serious enough to seek immediate medical attention from her primary physician and a pulmonary doctor. The diagnosis included small airways dysfunction syndrome. She was unresponsive to bronchodilators. She was positive for methacholine test, suggesting the development of asthma.

20.2.3.5 Employee 5

Amanda is a 49-year-old Caucasian woman with a history of asthma and allergies that required immunotherapy. However, despite this, she was able to work and get on with her life without any physical discomfort. After her exposure to the pesticide at the bank, she developed organophosphate-induced acute toxic symptoms such as burning in the eyes and mouth, nasal congestion, shortness of breath, fatigue, wheezing, sore throat, and nonproductive cough. She required immediate medical treatment by her primary physician and a pulmonary specialist. The diagnosis included irritant-induced bronchospasm, bronchial asthma, and allergic rhinitis.

20.2.4 Evidence that Excessive Dursban Pro Was Sprayed at the Bank

Dr. Patrick Chang of Environ Health Consultants Inc. was asked by the president of the bank to measure the pesticide residue at the bank and to advise him about the possible levels of exposure of his employees to the pesticide. Dr. Chang's initial visit was five days after the spray and he subsequently visited on two more occasions. Each time, Dr. Chang took surface and air samples and analyzed by GC-MS for chlorpyrifos and other solvents. Dursban Pro contains 22.5% chlorpyrifos and 77.5% solvents and other materials. Dow

Chemical Company recommends a working solution of 0.25% for routine application and 0.5% solution for heavy infestation. Representatives of the exterminating company thought that they used a 0.25% solution at the bank. However, analysis of the pesticide residue at the bank showed that too much Dursban was sprayed. Dr. Chang very rightly concluded that there could not have been a smell after 5 days if the recommended concentration of Dursban was sprayed. The analytical results showed that mistakes were made during the application of Dursban Pro. The wallpaper also contained chlorpyrifos residue even after 5 months. Thus, it can be concluded that excessive Dursban Pro spray caused serious health problems in employees of the bank. The conclusions drawn by Dr. Chang after the analysis of surface and air samples at the bank confirmed that the employees were exposed to excessive amounts of chlorpyrifos, which resulted in organophosphate toxicity (**4,12**).

20.2.5 Chlorpyrifos Toxicity

Dursban Pro contains chlorpyrifos and xylene, an organic solvent. Chlorpyrifos is a Class 3 toxic compound because it can cause irreversible effects that can be life threatening. It is an organophosphorus pesticide and is a white crystal-like solid with a strong odor. It does not mix well with water. Therefore, organic solvents are used before it is applied (**4,13**). An estimated 19 to 27 million pounds of chlorpyrifos are used in this country in agriculture and in households. As with any pesticide, improper use will result in its toxicity (**14**). Because of its extensive use, chlorpyrifos is a major source of exposure to pesticide in Americans and its exposure appears to be increasing with increase in its use. Exposure to chlorpyrifos can occur orally, though inhalation, or by absorption through the skin. Animal studies in the laboratory revealed that this pesticide is rapidly absorbed through the skin in a matter of minutes (**4**). It is likely that the employees at the bank were exposed mostly by inhalation and to some extent through the skin. Acute toxicity of this pesticide may cause headache, dizziness, loss of coordination, muscle twitching, tremors, nausea, vomiting, abdominal cramps, diarrhea, general weakness, blurred vision, pulmonary problems, wheezing, excessive perspiration, respiratory failure, and difficulty in breathing. Long-term effects may include neurological problems such as headaches, muscle weakness, confusion, and depression. Several cases of chlorpyrifos toxicity were reported from time to time. Eight people developed peripheral neuropathy after exposure to Dursban; five experienced memory loss and cognitive slowing (**15**). Five occupants of an office building showed toxic effects of chlorpyrifos. The pattern of symptoms suggests redistribution of the active organophosphate after absorption to a second body compartment with subsequent slow release of the still active substance into the bloodstream (**16**). Delayed effects may be produced after initial recovery. In the case of office workers reported above, even though the pesticide was applied outside, the office workers inside suffered toxic effects suggesting that the pesticide was drawn in through the air vents. Chlorpyrifos can cause permanent neurological damage including paralysis. Chlorpyrifos is known to decrease immune function and result in allergic reaction (17). Because of the continued reports of chlorpyrifos poisoning cases, the EPA has now prohibited all residential uses of foggers and broadcast products, all direct-application pet products including sprays, shampoos, and dips, and high concentrated product use on plants (17).

20.2.6 Conclusions

1. The acute, chronic, delayed, and long-lasting health effects of the five employees were caused by Dursban Pro pesticide that was sprayed in the bank.
2. Pesticide residue analysis at the bank unequivocally suggested that exterminators sprayed excessive concentrations of Dursban Pro pesticide.
3. This unfortunate accident was caused by a mistake in dilution of the concentrate solution.
4. The excessive amounts sprayed resulted in chemical sensitization, triggering the induction of new health problems and flare-up of existing health problems in the employees of the bank.
5. The negligence of the extermination company caused pain and suffering to the five women employed by the bank.

20.3 Chloroform Burns in the Mouth of a Dental Patient

20.3.1 Legal Aspects: Negligent Dentist and Burns in the Mouth

This case is about Ms. Peggy Masaro, who went to a dentist for a root canal procedure. While performing the root canal procedure, the dentist spilled chloroform in her mouth causing burns and tissue necrosis. This required tissue grafting in her mouth. She brought a civil lawsuit for monetary compensation against the dentist for professional negligence, which caused pain and suffering.

20.3.2 Medical Aspects: Chloroform Burns

Chloroform is a volatile organic solvent that is no longer used as an anesthetic. However, it is still used in dentistry during root canal procedures with gutta-percha cones. Chloroform is known to induce chemical burns in soft tissue areas, causing tissue necrosis. Chloroform is classified as a carcinogen.

20.3.3   Factual Background

Ms. Peggy Masaro is a 32-year-old Caucasian female, in good health who went to Dr. Thomas Serbin on February 24, 1999 seeking treatment for dental problems. The dentist suggested two options: extraction or root canal. The patient opted for root canal and Dr. Serbin performed this on March 9, 1999. The procedure included filling a cavity with Sealopex and #40 Gutta Percha. A day later, the patient complained that her jaw and gums hurt. The dentist told the patient that the area around tooth hurt due to accidental splashing of chloroform. The patient subsequently went to the emergency department at Repallo Hospital on March 12, 1999 seeking treatment for her pain in the gums and the jaw. According to Dr. Brian Krunz of the Emergency Department, on examination the patient exhibited a chemical burn along the buccal aspect of the gingiva just below the right lower canine/bicuspid area. The patient was given 2% Lidocaine to relieve her pain. Because of the persistent pain and increase in the necrotic area due to biting, the patient went to the School of Dental Medicine at the University of Plottsburg. The dentist there noted swelling of the lymph nodes, clicking in the temporomandibular joint, and sloughing and necrosis in the gingival margin around her tooth. The treatment suggested included soft tissue grafting and root canal retreatment. She subsequently contacted Drs. Somani and Quinsey for treatment. She underwent soft tissue grafting.

20.3.4   Chloroform in Dentistry

Dentists use gutta-percha cones as root-filling material in root canal work and chloroform is used as a solvent to soften the gutta-percha cones (**18**). However, due to a ban by the Food and Drug Administration on the use of chloroform in drugs and cosmetics, there has been some debate and concern about the use of chloroform in dentistry (**19**). Because of the safety concerns to dentists as well as patients, alternative and safe solvents as softening agents for gutta-percha cones are being explored (**20,21**). The uptake of chloroform by gutta-percha cones depends on the dipping time (**22**). An experienced dentist is aware of the chronic and acute toxicity of chloroform and is extremely careful in the use of chloroform in his or her dental practice. Normally such chemical burns to patients are quite rare. However, a spill of chloroform and subsequent chemical burn, and severe tissue necrosis resulting in the soft tissue graft is indicative of negligence by Dr. Thomas Serbin.

20.3.5   Chloroform and Cancer

First prepared in 1831, chloroform was initially employed as an ideal anesthetic. Later, acute and chronic toxicity of chloroform was discovered. The

National Cancer Institute has classified chloroform as a carcinogen in laboratory rodents (23). A significantly greater number of tumors were noticed in rats that were given chloroform in drinking water throughout their lifetime (24). The Environmental Protection Agency became concerned when it was discovered that chlorination of drinking water generates chloroform and other chlorinated hydrocarbons (25,26). Besides these public health concerns, chloroform has acute toxicity. Chloroform causes liver cell necrosis (27). Necrosis and subsequent compensatory cell proliferation are the ideal conditions to cause cancer. Acute chloroform tissue injury, necrosis, and compensatory cell regeneration are known to cause cancer by non-genotoxic mechanism (28,29). This was unequivocally confirmed by experiments conducted in rodents where histology and cellular regeneration index confirmed that tumors develop in areas where there was necrosis and cell regeneration (30,31).

20.3.6   Conclusions

Based on the available evidence and information from the published literature, it can be concluded with a reasonable degree of scientific certainty that:

1. Spilling of chloroform in Ms. Peggy Masaro's mouth during a root canal procedure by the dentist amounts to professional negligence.
2. Ms. Peggy Masaro suffered severe chloroform burns resulting in tissue necrosis, which subsequently required additional procedures and tissue grafting.
3. Dr. Thomas Serbin bears full responsibility for the pain and suffering caused to Ms. Peggy Masaro.

20.4   Do Not Eat Those Brownies

20.4.1   Legal Aspects: Brownies Laced with Ex-Lax

This case involves Steven Tesah, who was fired by the plant manager of Powdered Metals, Inc. Steven made brownies laced with Ex-Lax and made sure that his supervisor, Bill Feelicks, ate them. Steven complained to his union that it was a prank and he never intended to harm Mr. Feelicks; therefore, he should be reinstated. The plant manager says this action by Steven cannot be condoned as it amounts to a chemical assault. At the request of the union, the case went to binding arbitration.

20.4.2   Medical Aspects: Toxicity of Sennosides

The sennoside is an anthroquinone glucoside and is obtained from dried leaflets and pods of the Senna plant. Preparations made with sennosides are used as laxatives. Most of the time these stimulant laxatives are safe when taken in recommended doses. Large doses are toxic and cause adverse reactions in certain individuals. Bill Feelicks suffered toxic effects of sennosides by eating brownies laced with Ex-Lax tablets.

20.4.3   Factual Background

This case involves Steven Tesah, who was fired by the plant manager of Powdered Metals, Inc. because he made brownies laced with Ex-Lax and made sure that his supervisor, Bill Feelicks, ate them. The plant manager felt that Steven's actions were a chemical assault on Bill Feelicks.

This incident happened on the night of Tuesday, January 19, 1999, and Wednesday morning of January 20, 1999. Steven Tesah says he laced the brownies with Ex-Lax because he suspected that Bill Feelicks was stealing the workers' lunches and he wanted to teach Bill a lesson.

According to the plant manager, Steven became disgruntled when Bill wrote up Steven for not wearing a safety hat. To get back at Bill, Steven made brownies laced with Ex-Lax tablets. Ex-Lax is an over-the-counter laxative. It was stated that Steven made 12 brownies and mixed them with four Ex-Lax tablets. Based on the serious toxic reaction Bill suffered after eating the brownies, it was determined that Steven added much more than four Ex-Lax tablets. Bill went home from work at 7:00 p.m. and got sick immediately. He developed cramps, nausea, diarrhea, sleeplessness, and a run-down feeling for the next 12 to 14 hours.

It became apparent from the investigation that Steven targeted Bill because Steven warned other co-workers at the plant not to eat the brownies.

The plant manager asked custodial staff to retrieve the leftover brownies from the garbage. He sent the brownies to the local police department for testing. Bill's urine was collected and sent to a lab for analysis; however, the results are not available. The brownies retrieved from the garbage were sent to the Laboratory of International Toxy Services Inc. for toxicological analysis. The first laboratory report was incorrect as it was looking for phenolphthalein, the active ingredient in Ex-Lax. However, FDA banned the use of phenolphthalein in 1997 as a laxative in view of its carcinogenicity in rodents. Consequently, Ex-Lax was reformulated to contain docusate sodium, a stool softener, and sennosides, a laxative (4). Subsequent lab reports detected sennosides by thin layer chromatography, confirming that the brownies were indeed laced with Ex-Lax.

20.4.4   Toxicity of Sennosides

As noted earlier, Ex-Lax contains docusate sodium, sennosides, and other inactive ingredients (4). The sennoside is an anthroquinone glucoside, with a molecular weight 862.72 **(32)**. Sennosides are obtained from dried leaflets and pods of the Senna plant **(33,34)**. The recommended daily adult dose is 12 to 17 mg taken at bedtime **(4)**. Even though it is an over-the-counter medication, it is generally taken with the consent of a qualified physician. Most of the time stimulant laxatives are safe when taken in the recommended doses. However, as with all other medications, sennosides can give adverse reactions in certain individuals. The adverse reactions include abdominal pain, discomfort, diarrhea, nausea, and electrolyte and fluid imbalance. Large doses are toxic and are known to cause hepatitis and nephritis **(4,33)**. High doses of sennosides caused death in rats due to extensive loss of water and electrolytes following massive diarrhea **(34)**.

Bill Feelicks went home at approximately 7:00 p.m. and got sick afterward. He suffered cramps, sleeplessness, and a run-down feeling. In addition to severe cramps, he suffered severe diarrhea for 12 to 14 hours. These symptoms suggest that Bill's intake of Ex-Lax was several times the recommended daily dose and, consequently, he suffered severe toxicity of sennosides.

It can be concluded with a reasonable degree of scientific certainty that:

1. Bill had severe toxicity of sennosides resulting in intestinal cramps, diarrhea, nausea, and a run-down feeling.
2. Even a qualified and board-certified physician cannot prescribe a medication without the consent of the patient. Medical ethics and the law dictate that the patient's consent must be obtained before administering a drug.
3. Targeting an individual with Ex-Lax is a clear violation of medical ethics.
4. It is clearly a case of assault.

20.5 Toxic Anti-Gel Fumes and Asthma

20.5.1 Legal Aspects: Exposure to Anti-Gel Fumes and Development of Asthma

This case is about a senior high school student Jackie Rosemary, who alleges that she was forced to sit at the back of the school bus where she was exposed to the noxious fumes released from a canister containing diesel anti-gel. As a result, she developed severe asthma. She is suing the school district and the Chitti Kitti School Bus Company for violating the rules of the school district for transporting toxic canisters. She is demanding monetary compensation for her pain and suffering as she developed severe asthma.

20.5.2   Medical Aspects: Toxicity of Volatile Hydrocarbon Fumes

Diesel anti-gel contains aliphatic petroleum distillate (57 to 58%), aromatic petroleum distillate (19 to 20%), and aromatic hydrocarbon solvent mixture (20 to 21%). Acute inhalation of hydrocarbon vapors can result in exacerbation of an individual's asthma resulting in long-term health problems (**35**).

20.5.3   Factual Background

Jackie Rosemary is an 18-year-old Caucasian female. On February 28, 1995, she boarded a school bus at 7:05 to go to Portersville Christian School. She could not sit in her assigned seat in the last row because boxes of diesel anti-gel were stored there. She was directed to sit in another seat, which was directly in front of the boxes. At least four canisters in the boxes had broken seals and one canister was dented on the top. The diesel anti-gel leaked out from these canisters and the bottom of the box was saturated with the diesel anti-gel. Consequently, there was an unbearable smell due to diesel anti-gel fumes and several students, including the plaintiff, complained to the bus driver. The bus driver refused to let them open the bus windows because it was a very cold day. Jackie was exposed to vapors of the diesel anti-gel for more than 1 hour. She became sick and developed a cough, shortness of breath, headache, watery eyes, and nausea. As soon as the bus reached the school, Jackie went to the school office and reported the incident. She telephoned her mother to pick her up and take her home. The school nurse was not there.

The plaintiff's health problems started subsequent to her exposure to the vapors of diesel anti-gel in the bus. The plaintiff had mild asthma before the incident and after the incident, she developed persistent cough, breathing difficulties, and wheezing. Her condition worsened from mild asthma to high-grade asthma. The plaintiff was taken to Dr. Peng Cheng Ming, an expert in treating lung diseases. He is board certified in pulmonary medicine and critical care medicine. According to Dr. Ming's deposition testimony, the plaintiff had asthma going back to her childhood and was limited to only one or two asthma attacks per year, which were managed by a nonsteroidal inhaler, Proventil. Dr. Ming concluded that because of her exposure to dangerous vapors in the school bus, there was an exacerbation of her asthma requiring a prolonged course of oral steroids. Based on his long years of clinical practice, Dr. Ming concluded that hydrocarbons present in diesel anti-gel are bronchial irritants, which caused chronic symptoms similar to reactive airways dysfunction syndrome (RADS). Dr. Ramakant Joshi, who also examined Jackie, disagreed with the opinion of Dr. Ming, and said that Jackie was normal and had mild symptoms of asthma consistent with the results of lung function studies. Dr. Ming reiterated that just because the lung function of the plaintiff was normal on a particular day does not mean she did not have asthma because asthma is an episodic disease and can be unpredictable. There is ample clinical and experimental evidence to support Dr. Ming's conclusions. The plaintiff's attorney contends that the undisputed facts as they unfold were as follows:

- The defendants violated the law and transported the dangerous diesel anti-gel cans in the back of the school bus when students were riding on the bus.
- The box contained cans of diesel anti-gel with broken seals that were subjected to bumps and shakes of the bus ride resulting in spillage of their contents.
- The plaintiff was exposed to dangerous and noxious vapors of the diesel anti-gel.
- The plaintiff's pulmonary physician concluded that Jackie was sensitized by the noxious vapors, which resulted in exacerbation of her asthma and consequently she developed persistent and long-term health problems.

20.5.4   Toxicity of Diesel Anti-Gel

Diesel anti-gel, product code M22-16, manufactured by Automax Company, is added to diesel fuel to prevent it from freezing in cold weather. This product contains aliphatic petroleum distillate (57 to 58%), aromatic petroleum distillate (19 to 20%), and aromatic hydrocarbon solvent mixture (20 to 21%). Published literature clearly shows that low viscosity hydrocarbons present in diesel anti-gel are aspiration hazards. These vapors have acute and chronic toxicity. Acute exposure can cause headache, nausea, watery eyes, and in severe cases even death. Pulmonary damage, transient CNS depression, and chronic lung dysfunction can occur.

20.5.5   Chemical Sensitization, Allergic Reactions, and Asthma

Human and animal data suggest that these volatile hydrocarbons may induce or aggravate asthma in susceptible individuals (36). As stated previously, in addition to acute toxicity, persistent exposure leads to chronic toxicity. Moreover, in susceptible individuals, chemical sensitization leads to chronic respiratory effects and physician-diagnosed asthma (37). Intermittent complaints of eye irritation, nausea, and headache were associated with exposure to gasoline vapors (38). In susceptible individuals, small amounts of low viscosity hydrocarbons aspirated over a large portion of the pulmonary bed can result in chemical pneumonitis and respiratory distress. Vapors of highly volatile hydrocarbons are highly lipid soluble and therefore are well absorbed through the lungs with distribution to the brain and other organs (**39**). Such lipid-soluble chemical irritants, once absorbed, distribute to at least two body compartments. The irritants in one compartment are cleared resulting in the disappearance of symptoms but the chemical irritant stored in lipid depots can result in persistent and chronic health problems (**40**).

An appreciation and familiarity with immunotoxicology scientific literature suggests that even small doses can result in chemical sensitization in susceptible individuals. It appears that inhalation exposure can produce asthma by several mechanisms. Sensitization with the production of IgE specific for a substance can lead to symptoms on re-exposure via most cell degranulation and the release of inflammatory mediators. Respiratory irritants can lead to asthma and rhinitis through interaction with chemical irritant receptors in the airway. The reactive airways syndrome is a chronic asthma-like syndrome resulting from a single exposure to a respiratory irritant. An acute exposure to a respiratory irritant can cause chronic asthma with persistent bronchial hyperactivity that continues long after the toxic exposure. It is no wonder that people with asthma react even to small doses of chemical irritant as their airways are hyper-responsive to a number of chemical irritants (**41,42**).

Why do people with asthma show immediate and delayed symptoms on exposure to chemical irritants? In experimental asthma triggered by chemical irritants, two distinct phases are observed. The immediate phase occurs within a short period of time, which may resolve spontaneously or with treatment, followed by a late phase, which occurs later and may persist for a long time (**43,44**).

Allergic reactions could be defined as the adverse reactions that lead to tissue damage. Sometimes these allergic reactions can have fatal consequences due to specific immune responses usually to exogenous antigens. In the context of toxicology, allergic reaction resulting from immune responses to chemicals and drugs are of greatest relevance. These allergic reactions can lead to severe asthma due to the exposed chemicals producing IgE to cause hypersensitivity reactions in the respiratory tract (**45**).

20.5.6 Comments on Toxicology Report Submitted by the Defendant's Attorney

The defendant's attorney obtained a toxicology report from Dr. Hitori Fujusava, an internist. There are several issues raised in this report that warrant comment.

1. *Observation*: Jackie's exposure would be classified as short term and sub-acute.

Comment: Jackie sat directly in front of the canisters with broken seals and was exposed to the vapors of diesel anti-gel for nearly 80 minutes. Her exposure was substantial as revealed by her immediate symptoms. She developed headache, nausea, eye irritation, cough, and shortness of breath. It was fortunate that she did not die.

2. *Observation*: Instead of seeking immediate medical help, she called her mother on the day of the incident.

   Comment: The school nurse comes one day a week for only a few hours and was not present on the day of the incident. Jackie's mother is a qualified registered nurse. What medical help would the school nurse give that Jackie's mother could not give?

3. *Observation*: The bus door opened and closed several times for students to disembark. With the opening and closing of school bus door, the concentration of fumes would change during the 80-minute bus ride.

   Comment: The fumes were in the back of the bus and the driver operated the door in the front of the bus. Opening and closing this door was not going to change the concentration of the vapors in the back of the bus. An industrial hygienist or an occupational safety engineer can substantiate this possibility.

20.5.7 Conclusions

It can be concluded with a reasonable degree of scientific certainty that:

1. Jackie was exposed to diesel anti-gel vapors for 80 minutes.
2. This exposure caused exacerbation of her mild asthma to develop into high-degree asthma.
3. Thus, the plaintiff suffered and continues to suffer chronic and long-term asthma requiring the use of steroid medications with dangerous and potentially harmful side effects.
4. The school and the bus company broke the law and subjected Jackie to intense exposure to toxic diesel anti-gel vapors.
5. The damage done to Jackie's health appears to be chronic and long lasting and was a direct result of this exposure.

20.6 Negligent Pharmacist and Drug Overdose

20.6.1 Legal Aspects: Pharmacy Negligence and Drug Overdose

This case deals with an unintentional overdose of fentanyl and its toxic effects on Andrew Beller. Mr. Beller suffered serious toxic effects of fentanyl due to a mistake made in writing the wrong instructions on the filled prescription. He had to be rushed to the emergency room of a local hospital and was at the hospital for several days. This mistake resulted in missing work for which he lost his job. He filed a civil lawsuit for monetary compensation against the pharmacist and the Chandra Drugstore Corporation.

20.6.2 Medical Aspects: Professional Negligence and Drug Toxicity

Duragesic patch contains fentanyl, which is well suited for transdermal administration because of its lipid solubility, high potency, and low molecular weight. Fentanyl is extremely lipophilic. This transdermal system is useful in the treatment of malignant and nonmalignant chronic pain. This drug is oftentimes abused and has serious side effects. Several deaths have been reported. Fentanyl is not detected by routine urine drug screen, so the total number of deaths that occur due to fentanyl overdose may be seriously underestimated. Fentanyl's side effects include sedation, nausea, vomiting, and constipation.

20.6.3 Factual Background

This report deals with an unintentional overdose of fentanyl and its toxic effects on Andrew Beller, a Caucasian male, 54 years of age. He suffers from pain secondary to a spinal cord injury. He also has a history of Crohn's disease. He admits to cigarette smoking and denies alcohol use. He is under the care of his primary care physician and a neurologist for the management of pain. He was on pain medications. He was asked to apply Duragesic 100 mg patch by his doctor. This prescription was filled at Chandra Drugs. The pharmacy filled the prescription and gave him the Duragesic patch with erroneous written instructions that the patch should be applied once every three hours. Mr. Beller followed these written instructions and applied the Duragesic patch once every three hours. Actually, the therapeutic recommendation is that the Duragesic patch be applied once every three days. Because of this, Mr. Beller overdosed and suffered severe toxicity of fentanyl. His friends found him lethargic and unconscious and called his mother immediately. His mother found her son lying on the bed, unresponsive. She had difficulty waking him. Soon, paramedics were called in and they brought him to the emergency department of the Marsburgh Research Hospital. It was concluded by the doctors at the emergency department that Mr. Beller was exhibiting the symptoms of narcotic overdose. Mr. Beller had mental status changes. There was concern for GI bleeding. He had abnormal cardiac enzymes. He had nausea, vomiting, and edema of the lower extremities. He had decreased renal function secondary to fentanyl toxicity. Subsequent to his discharge from the Marsburgh Research Hospital, he continued to suffer the toxic effects of fentanyl. He visited Core Hospital, where it was documented that he suffered from fatigue, nausea, vomiting, confusion, CNS depression, slowed breathing and heartbeat, and loss of consciousness. He was fortunate that he did not die due to fentanyl toxicity.

20.6.4   Fentanyl

Fentanyl is a synthetic narcotic analgesic of high potency and short duration. This drug has been in clinical use since 1963 as an adjunct to surgical anesthesia often in combination with nitrous oxide. It can be administered intravenously, injected, or as an intradermal patch for the management of pain. On a weight-by-weight basis, it is 50 to 100 times more potent than morphine. Fentanyl is extremely lipophilic, more so than any other currently available opiates. This drug is oftentimes abused and has serious side effects. Several deaths have been reported. Fentanyl is not detected by routine urine drug screen, so the total number of deaths that occur might be seriously underestimated. Fentanyl side effects include sedation, nausea, vomiting, and constipation. This drug can cause rigidity in the chest wall muscle resulting in a condition known as "wooden chest syndrome." Loss of consciousness, respiratory depression, and CNS depression also occur. Fentanyl side effects have the potential to cause discomfort, injury, and death in patients. The overdose effects are respiratory depression, bradycardia, hypotension, hypertension, miosis, mydriasis, and dystonic reaction (**46-49**). Fentanyl toxicity can result in depressed renal function (**50,51**).

20.6.5   Transdermal Fentanyl Patch

Fentanyl is well suited for transdermal administration because of its lipid solubility, high potency, and low molecular weight. Transdermal fentanyl forms within the upper skin layers before entering microcirculation. Therapeutic blood levels are attained in approximately 12 to 16 hours after applying the patch. The drug decreases slowly, with a half-life of 16 to 22 hours following patch removal. These properties make it possible for therapeutic doses of fentanyl to be absorbed through relatively small areas of the skin. This noninvasive transdermal system releases fentanyl up to 72 hours. The fentanyl levels remain in circulation for 72 hours after initiation and thereafter remain stable with repeated administration every three days (**52**).This delivery system, brand name Duragesic, is manufactured by Janssen Pharmaceuticals and has been in use in the United States since 1991.

The most serious and life threatening side effects occur when an individual overdoses on this medication. Hundreds of deaths have been linked to overdose of the fentanyl patch (**7-9**). In response to these reports, the

FDA issued a public health advisory in July 2005 (updated in 2007) and Janssen Pharmaceuticals, the maker of Duragesic fentanyl patch updated the label and warned health care professionals and their patients about the serious and oftentimes fatal side effects that may occur because of overdose (53–55).

Health care professionals including doctors and pharmacists are expected to know that once the Duragesic patch is placed on the skin of the patient, it is slowly absorbed from the skin into the bloodstream and steady state drug levels are reached by 72 hours. By renewing the patches every 72 hours, the steady state drug levels are maintained. If used properly, it is effective in controlling pain in cancer and non-cancerous patients. Fentanyl continues to be absorbed into the systemic circulation even after the patch has been removed. This delayed action of the drug after transdermal application has clinical and toxicological consequences (52).

It is the responsibility of the pharmacy to instruct the patient in the proper use of the Duragesic patch; otherwise, overdose of fentanyl can result leading to serious side effects such as sweating, nausea, vomiting, confusion, diarrhea, nervousness, hallucinations, breathing problems, CNS and depression, and bradycardia. Several fatalities have been reported due to fentanyl overdose (55,56).

20.6.6 Conclusions

Based on the available evidence from published literature, it can be concluded with a reasonable degree of medical and scientific certainty that:

1. Mr. Beller suffered several serious side effects of fentanyl toxicity due to the use of Duragesic patch.
2. Mr. Beller followed the written instructions of the pharmacy and applied the Duragesic patch once every 3 hours as instructed.
3. The pharmacy was careless and negligent when it instructed Mr. Beller to apply the Duragesic patches once every 3 hours instead of once every 3 days.
4. The Chandra Drugstore, which filled the prescription, is solely responsible for the pain and suffering caused to Mr. Beller.

References

1. Cornell University Law School. Tort law: an overview. http://topics.law.cornell.edu/wex/tort.
2. What is tort law? http://wisegeek.com/what-is-tort-law.htm.
3. Wikipedia. Tort. http://en.wikipedia.org/wiki/Tort.
4. Clinical Information, Health Care Series, Micromedix Inc. 1999.

5. Hodgson, M.J., Block, G.D., and Parkinson, D.K. Organophosphorus poisoning in office workers. *J. Occupational Med.* **28**:434–437, 1986.

6. Kopsyc, Z. and Strehl, M. Acute parapsoriasis in a 5-year-old girl. *Wiad Lek.* **43**:308–311, 1990.

7. Matsushita, T., Aoyama, K., Yoshimi, K., Fujita, Y., and Ueda, A. Allergic contact dermatitis from organophosphorus insecticides. *Industrial Health* **23**:145–153, 1985.

8. Stoianov, B.G., Federov, S.M., Selisskii, G.D., Agakishiev, D.D., and Alchangian, L.V. Measures for the combined therapy and prevention of dermatoses occurring in workers in contact with organophosphorus pesticides. *Vestn. Dermatol. Venerol.* **7**:29–34, 1989.

9. Lotti, T., Ghersetich, I., Commacchi, C., and Jorizzo, J.L. Cutaneous small-vessel vasculitis. *J. Am. Acad. Dermatol.* **39**:667–687, 1998.

10. Kuby, J. Leukocyte migration and inflammation. In: *Immunology.* Goldsby, R.A., Kindt, T.J., and Osborne, B.A., Eds. W.H. Freeman and Co., New York, 1997, chap. 15.

11. Thrasher, J.D., Madison, R., and Broughton, A. Immunologic abnormalities in humans exposed to chlorpyrifos: Preliminary observations. *Arch. Environ. Health* **48**:89–93, 1993.

12. Weyel, D.A. Occupational Health Consultants, Inc. Carnegie, PA. Letter to Mr. Larry L. Travis, President, United National Bank, Moundsville, WV. Re: Dursban Measurements at United National Bank. October 2, 1996, October 15, 1996, and March 4, 1997.

13. Chlorpyrifos. CAS # 2921-88-2, TOX FAOs, September 1997.

14. Barlo, D.M. Memorandum. Recent Activities Concerning Chlorpyrifos. USEPA, January 29, 1997.

15. Kaplan, J.G., Kessler, J., Rosenberg, N., Pack, D., and Schaumburg, H.H. Sensory neuropathy associated with Dursban (chlorpyrifos) exposure. *Neurology* **43**:2193–2196, 1993.

16. Thrasher, J.D., Madison, R., and Broughton, A. Immunologic abnormalities in humans exposed to chlorpyrifos: Preliminary observations. *Arch. Environ. Health* **48**:89–93, 1993.

17. Headquarters Press Release. Agreement reached between EPA and Chlorpyrifos pesticide registrants. USEPA, June 6, 1997. www.epa.gov/ncer/childrenscenters/full_text/33919.pdf

18. Allard, U. and Anderson, L. Exposure of dental personnel to chloroform in root-filling procedures. *Endodod. Dent. Traumatol.* **8**:155–159, 1992.

19. McDonald, M.N. and Vire, D.E. Chloroform in the endodontic operatory. *J. Endodod.* **18**:301–313, 1992.

20. Wilcox, L.R. Endodontic retreatment with halothane versus chloroform solvent. *J. Endodod.* **21**:305–307, 1995.

21. Zakariasen, K.L., Brayton, S.M., and Collison, D.M. Efficient and effective root canal retreatment without chloroform. *J. Can. Dent. Assoc.* **56**:509–512, 1990.

22. Margelos, J., Verdelis, K., and Eliades, G. Chloroform uptake by gutta-percha and assessment of its concentration during chloroform-dip technique. *J. Endodod.* **22**:547–550, 1996.

23. Winslow, S.G. and Gerstner, H.B. Health aspects of chloroform—a review. *Drug Chem. Toxicol.* **1**:259–275, 1978.

24. Tumasonis, C.F., McMartin, D.N., and Bush, B. Toxicity of chloroform and bromochlormethane when administered over a lifetime in rats. *J. Envviron. Pathol. Toxicol.* **7**:55–63, 1987.

25. Dunnick, J.K. and Melnick, R.L. Assessment of the carcinogenic potential of chlorinated water: experimental studies of chlorine, chloramine, and trihalomethanes. *J. Natl. Cancer Inst.* **85**:817–822, 1993.

26. Wigle, D.T. Safe drinking water: a public health challenge. *Chronic. Dis. Can.* **19**:103–107, 1998.

27. Rao, K.N., Virji, M.A., Moraca, M.A., Diven, W.F., Martin, T.G., and Shneider, S.M. Role of serum markers for liver function and regeneration in the management of chloroform poisoning. *J. Anal. Toxicol.* **17**:99–102, 1993.

28. Butterworth, B.E., Templin, M.V., Borghoff, S.J., Conolly, R.B., Kedderis, G.L., and Wolf, D.C. The role of regenerative cell proliferation in chloroform-induced cancer. *Toxicol. Lett.* **82-83**:23–26, 1995.

29. Kegelmeeyer, A.E., Sprankle, C.S., Horesovsky, G.J., and Butterworth, B.E. Differential display identified changes in mRNA levels in regenerating livers from chloroform treated mice. *Mol. Carcinog.* **20**:288–297, 1997.

30. Golden, R.J., Holm, S.E., Robinson, D.E., Julkunen, P.H., and Reese, E.A. Chloroform mode of action: implications for cancer risk assessment. *Regul. Toxicol. Pharmacol.* **26**:142–155, 1997.

31. Reitz, R.H., Fox, T.R., and Quast, J.F. Mechanistic considerations for carcinogenic risk estimation: chloroform. *Environ. Health Perspect.* **46**:163–168, 1988.

32. Gilman, A.G., Goodman, L.S., Rall, T.W., and Murad, F. (Eds.). *Goodman and Gilman's The Pharmacological Basis of Therapeutics.* Macmillan Publishing Co., New York, 1985, 1000–1001.

33. Franz, G. The senna drug and its chemistry. *Pharmacol.* **47**:2–6, 1993.

34. Mengs, U. Toxic effects of sennosides in laboratory animals and *in vitro*. *Pharmacol.* **36**:180–187, 1988.

35. Windholtz, M. (Ed.). *The Merck Index.* Merck & Co, Rahway, NJ, 1976.

36. Rodriguez de la Vega, A., Casaco, A., Garcia, M. et al. Kerosene-induced asthma. *Ann. Allergy* **64**:362–363, 1990.

37. Kullman, G.T. and Hill, R.A. Indoor air quality affected by abandoned gasoline tanks. *Appl. Occup. Environ. Hyg.* **5**:36–37, 1990.

38. Linden, C.H. Volatile substances of abuse. *Emerg. Med. Clin. N. Am.* **8**:559–578, 1990.

39. Meggs, W.J. RADS and RUDS. The toxic induction of asthma and rhinitis. *Clin. Toxicol.* **32**:487–501, 1994.

40. Brooks, S.M., Weiss, M.A., and Berstein, I.L. Reactive airways dysfunction syndrome. Case reports of persistent asthma syndrome after high level of irritant exposure. *Chest* **88**:376–384, 1985.

41. Lemanske, R.F. and Kaliner, M.A. Late phase allergic reactions. In: *Allergy: Principles and Practice*, 4th ed. Middleton Jr., E., Reed, C.E., Ellis, E.F. et al., Eds. Mosby, St. Louis, MO, 1993, 320–361.

42. Kimber, I., Gerberick, G.F., van Loveren, H., and House, R.V. Chemical allergy: Molecular mechanism and practical applications. *Fundam. Appl. Toxicol.* **19**:479–483, 1992.

43. Ohta, K., Yamashita, N., Tajima, M., Miyasaka, T., Nakano, J., Nakajima, H., Ishii, A., Horiuchi, T., Mano, K., and Miyamoto, T. Diesel exhaust particulate induces airway hyper responsiveness in a murine model: Essential role of GM-CSF. *J. Allergy Clin. Immunol.* **104**:1024–1030, 1999.
44. Miyabara, Y., Ichinose, T., Takano, H., Lim, H., and Sagai, M. Effect of diesel exhaust on allergic airway inflammation in mice. *J. Allergy Clin. Immunol.* **102**:805–812, 1998.
45. Nel, A.E., Diaz-Sanchez, D., Ng, D., Hiura, T., and Saxon, A. Enhancement of allergic inflammation by the interaction between diesel exhaust particles and the immune system. *J. Allergy Clin. Immunol.* **102**:539–554, 1998.
46. Baselt, R.C. and Cravey, R.H. Fentanyl. In: *Disposition of Toxic Drugs and Chemicals in Man*, 4th ed. Chemical Toxicology Institute, Foster City, CA, 1995, 319–322.
47. Karch, S.B. Fentanyl. In: *Karch's Pathology of Drug Abuse*. CRC Press, Boca Raton, FL, 2001, 364–369.
48. Fentanyl/Dropeperidol. In: Poisindex. Micromedix Healthcare Series. www.online6.hsls.pitt.edu, 2006.
49. Duragesic. Guides to prescription drugs. Encyclopedia of Medicine.
50. Castiglia, Y.M., Braz, J.R., Vianna, P.T., Lemonica, L., and Vane, L.A. Effect of high dose of fentanyl on renal function in dogs. *Sao Paulo Med. J.* **115**:1433–1439, 1997.
51. Kornick, C.A., Santiago-Palma, J., Moryl, N., Pyne, R., and Obbens, E.A.M.T. Benefit-risk assessment of transdermal fentanyl for the treatment of chronic pain. *Drug Safety* **26**:951–973, 2003.
52. Fentanyl side effects. www.drugs.com/sfx/fentanyl-side-effects.html.
53. Duragesic patch recall. www.lawyersandsettlements.com, 2006.
54. Duragesic patch overdose lawyers. www.lawyers.com, 2006.
55. Fentanyl Transdermal System (marketed as Duragesic) Information. FDA Alert for Health Care Professionals. http://www.fda.gov/Drugs/DrugSafety/PostmarketDrugSafetyInformationforPatientsandProviders/ucm114961.htm.
56. Rosenthal, N. Important drug warning. Janssen Pharmaceuticals, Titusville, NJ, 2005.

Workers' Compensation 21

In this chapter, cases pertaining to workers' compensation are presented. Workers' compensation (also known as workers' comp or workman's comp in the United States or compo in Australia) provides compensation for workers injured on the job. This provides monetary compensation for replacement of wages and medical benefits of the employees. The employee agrees to relinquish further claims in a lawsuit against the employer for claims of negligence or tort. Workers' compensation laws differ from state to state and from country to country. In general, workers' compensation benefits provide a fixed monthly monetary income and health insurance. In the United States, workers' compensation law was first passed in Maryland in 1902. Now, instead of using the term workman's compensation, the gender-neutral term workers' compensation is used. In the United States, most employees who are injured on the job have an absolute right to medical care and monetary benefits. Such payments depend on the employee's temporary or permanent disability. The employer buys insurance from private insurance companies to pay for the employee's disability. Workers' compensation is administered on a state-by-state basis. The federal government pays its own workers' compensation benefits to its employees through regular appropriations. Workers' compensation laws not only cover injuries sustained by the employee on the job but also include work-related diseases. Usually a review board calculates the nature of the injury and the amount of compensation (1-4).

21.1 Toxicity of Aircraft Fuels

21.1.1 Legal Aspects: Loss of Immunity, and Amputation of Fingers and Lower Limbs

This case is about Mr. Bill Furguson, who worked as an aircraft maintenance technician at Vanholt Aircraft Company. He developed immune deficiency, severe infections, septic shock, and renal failure. He and his wife Mary allege that he was exposed to toxic aviation fuel fumes resulting in loss of immune function and other health problems, culminating in amputation of some of the fingers on both hands and bilateral amputation of the lower limbs. He is seeking monetary compensation for loss of his potential for employment.

211

21.1.2 Medical Aspects: Toxicity of Aviation Fuels

Jet fuels are toxic and the toxicity of jet fuels depends upon the level and duration of exposure. Mr. Furguson was exposed to jet fuel substantial enough to cause severe immune deficiency. The hydrocarbons and benzene in jet fuel are known to be immuno-toxic. Consequently, Mr. Furguson developed disseminated intra-vascular coagulopathy (DIC). He also developed gangrene in his feet and hands. His doctors concluded that the gangrene on his legs and hands were caused by his exposure to toxins at his job.

21.1.3 Factual Background

Mr. Bill Furguson is a 30-year-old Caucasian male. He is a high school graduate and had 2 years of college. He has been working as a lineman at Vanholt Aircraft Company for nearly 3 years until the day of his hospitalization and incapacitation due to severe infections and surgical interventions to amputate six fingers on both hands and both of his lower limbs. At present, he is totally disabled. Prior to this, he reports that he worked as a security guard in a prison and a service technician at Easy Go Rental Car Company for 2 years. He was also employed as stock clerk in a grocery store and worked in an amusement park.

At Vanholt Aircraft, he worked as a lineman and his job was to fill the aircraft with jet fuel. He was subsequently promoted as a training coordinator with the responsibility to train co-workers in fueling operations. He was dealing with jet fuel and 100-octane aviation gasoline called AV gas. These commercial jet fuels were a kerosene type and contained benzene, toluene, and other aliphatic and aromatic hydrocarbons. He pumped these fuels from the tankers to the aircraft. Sometimes, he had to de-fuel the aircraft based on passenger load. He was also responsible for pumping gasoline from the big underground storage tanks to the tanker trucks. He inhaled gasoline vapors constantly and sometimes the gasoline spilled on his hands and face and splashed onto his clothes. The employees were not provided with gloves. Many times, his shoes and socks got wet and saturated with gasoline. The soles of his shoes used to melt. He worked at Vanholt Aircraft for nearly three years until he was permanently disabled. Thus, he was chronically exposed to jet fuel and aviation gas. Mary Furguson reiterates that her husband's clothes smelled of gasoline when he came home from work. There is no evidence that the management of Vanholt Aircraft ever mentioned the levels of fuel to which the workers were exposed. There is no evidence to show that the workers were ever made aware of the constituents of jet fuel. They did not know that constituents of jet fuel such as kerosene, hydrocarbons, and benzene are quite toxic to humans, if exposed chronically at higher than threshold levels. These toxic exposures resulted in Mr. Furguson developing severe infection on March 5, 2000, which culminated in the amputation of his fingers and lower limbs. Thus, an active and healthy productive young man was reduced to a life of disability, long-term medical care, and dependence on others for his day-to-day care.

21.1.4   Medical History

Bill Furguson is married and lives with his wife Mary at her parents' house. Mr. Furguson's father and mother are living and have no apparent medical problems. His two brothers and two sisters are in good health. He does not smoke, drink alcohol, or do drugs. He had testicular cancer in 1986 and was treated with chemotherapy. He developed toxoplasmosis as a complication of chemotherapy. He is free of cancer and his health has been good thus far.

On March 5, 2000, he developed a fever of 103°F and complained that his feet were burning. He was dehydrated and his nose turned purple and blackish. He was taken to Good Health General Hospital. He was told that he probably had a viral infection, most probably flu, and was sent home. Later, his condition worsened. He was taken to the emergency room at The University of Radymond Medical Center Hospital. Due to the onset of severe infection, he developed septic shock and renal failure. The microbiology laboratory results showed that Mr. Furguson was infected with *Neisseria meningitides*. He developed disseminated intra-vascular coagulopathy (DIC). Because of blood clots, the blood supply was cut off to his tissues resulting in tissue necrosis. He developed gangrene in his feet and hands. His doctors concluded that the gangrenes on his legs and hands were caused by his exposure to toxins at his job. Amputation on his hands resulted in the removal of the index and long fingers on his right hand and the index finger, long finger, ring finger and pinkie finger on his left hand. He also underwent bilateral amputations of his lower limbs. *Neisseria meningitides* is a normal bacterium present in the throat in a normal healthy population. This does not grow virulently and cause infection unless immunity is compromised. Mr. Furguson is not diabetic. He was not on immunosuppressive drugs and had no cancer. Therefore, his immune deficiency was caused by his exposure to toxins in his job. Mr. Furguson is now completely disabled and he needs constant medical care.

21.1.5   Toxicity of Jet Fuel and Aviation Gasoline

Mr. Bill Furguson pumped jet fuel and aviation gas in refueling aircraft. Jet fuel is a complex mixture of hydrocarbons containing n-alkanes, branched alkanes, cycloparaffins, benzenes, alkylhenzeuns, and kerosene blends (5). It is an established fact that exposure to jet fuel can occur from both occupational and environmental sources. The sources of occupational exposures include transfer operations from or to storage tanks, tanker trucks, fueling aircraft, and filling, draining, and maintenance of fuel tanks. OSHA

214 Forensic Toxicology: Medico-Legal Case Studies

has estimated that 9730 employees were occupationally exposed to jet fuel between 1980 and 1983 (5). At that rate, many more workers may have been exposed up to the present day. The toxicity of jet fuel depends upon the level and duration of exposure. Therefore, Mr. Furguson was exposed to substantial jet fuel to cause severe immune deficiency. The hydrocarbons and the constituent benzene in jet fuel are known to be immunotoxic (5-15).

There are no OSHA guidelines for jet fuel exposure. However, the U.S. Naval Office has guidelines for jet fuel exposure. It is suggested that these exposures should not be more than an average of 350 mg/m^3 for 8 hours or 1000 mg/m^3 for 15 minutes. On the other hand, OSHA has strict guidelines for benzene exposure. Benzene was recognized as a human carcinogen 100 years ago and is known to have hematotoxicity. Consequently, OSHA recommends 1 ppm of benzene exposure (16). Some experts think that even this level should be reduced further. Benzene and other hydrocarbons in jet fuel cause immune deficiency resulting in a decrease in immune cells such as T suppressor cells, B-lymphocytes, and macrophages in peripheral blood thymus and spleen. The immuno-toxic effect of benzene was demonstrated in murine models besides the observation that workers exposed to benzene have serious immune deficiencies (16).

The animal studies demonstrated that inhalation of benzene vapors affects humeral and cell mediated immunity. The physicians treating Mr. Furguson felt that benzene caused systemic as well as local immune deficiency causing the gangrene in his hands and feet. Mr. Furguson also suffered colds and flu-like symptoms suggestive of exposure to hydrocarbon vapors and benzene. The fact that *Neisseria meningitides* is a normal bacterium in a healthy human population and the fact that Mr. Furguson who was otherwise healthy contracted this infection underscores that he developed immune deficiency due to exposure to jet fuel.

21.1.6 Conclusions

Review of hospital medical records of Mr. Furguson and the medical reports from physicians treating him underscore the fact that he was an active, healthy and productive young man until he suffered *Neisseria meningitidis* infection on March 5, 2000. It is also an established fact that this bacterium is present in the throat of normal healthy individuals and the immune surveillance system in the body keeps it in check. Normal healthy individuals are not infected with this bacterium. When the system fails, then this bacterium becomes virulent and grows unchecked causing massive infection resulting in morbid and oftentimes fatal consequences. Diabetes, immunosuppressive drugs, AIDS, and cancer can cause immunodeficiency, predisposing a person to infections. Mr. Furguson had none of these issues. Therefore, his infectious disease specialist and other clinicians treating him very rightly concluded that exposure to toxins at his workplace caused the infection. Based on the deposition statements of several physicians and their reports and based on medical and scientific literature, it can be concluded that:

1. Mr. Furguson's immune system was impaired due to his exposure to hydrocarbons and benzene in jet fuel at his workplace.
2. This infection resulted in DIC and blood clots cutting blood supply to the tissues. The tissues became necrotic and he went into septic shock and kidney failure.
3. Lack of blood supply and oxygen resulted in gangrene in his lower limbs, feet, and hands.
4. The consequence was amputation of six fingers on both hands and bilateral amputation of the lower limbs.
5. Thus, a productive, healthy young man became completely disabled requiring further reconstructive plastic surgeries, rehabilitation, and support from his loved ones.

21.2 Two-Car Collision and Death of a TV Station Executive

21.2.1 Legal Aspects: Two-Car Collision, Death

This case is about Mr. Donard Derry who died in a car collision. He was presumptive positive for blood alcohol, which was later found to be due to contamination from his stomach contents. Mrs. Derry brought a civil lawsuit for monetary compensation under workers' compensation law against the TV station where he was working at the time of his death. The TV station contends that the defendant was intoxicated and died in a road accident for which they are not responsible. Later, the TV station reached an out of court settlement with Mrs. Derry.

21.2.2 Medical Aspects: Presumptive DUI

In the case of a death due to a severe auto accident, the autopsy blood obtained from the chest cavity might be contaminated with unabsorbed alcohol from the stomach. For this reason, the presence of presumptive alcohol from the chest cavity needs to be checked with the alcohol present in blood obtained from other areas of the body.

21.2.3 Factual Background

This accident occurred on State Road YR 55 involving two cars resulting in one fatality. The accident happened on September 28, 2003 at 5:05 a.m.

Vehicle 1 was driven by Mr. Donard Derry. He was a Caucasian male, 36 years of age, 6 feet 1 inch tall and weighing 230 pounds. He was driving a silver 2000 Volvo station wagon, which collided with another vehicle and then hit a concrete pillar. The car sustained major front-end damage. The police arrived at the scene at 5:19 a.m. and found that the driver of the other car did not sustain injuries. He was let go from the scene of the accident. The police never investigated whether the driver of the second car was intoxicated with alcohol or drugs or whether there was any road rage involved in this accident. There were no other witnesses to the accident. When the police arrived at the accident site, an ambulance was already there. According to paramedics, Mr. Derry was unresponsive and found slumped over the passenger seat. The death certificate indicates that death was at 8:21 a.m. on September 28, 2003. How long Mr. Derry lived after the accident is not known and the time of death after the accident was not determined.

Mr. Derry was director of sales for TV, Xyz. As a director of sales, he was used to visiting several places of entertainment for promotion of upcoming events. He was at Kona Seema's until it closed at 3:30 a.m. Donard Derry came to Erra Matti nightclub at approximately 1:00 a.m., had a few drinks, and left. The roads were wet. Mr. Ravi Teja, another witness, saw Donard Derry at a traffic light at approximately 4:00 a.m. They talked from their cars through the open windows.

21.2.4 Autopsy

The autopsy on Donard Derry's body was conducted by Dr. Guru Singh, for Path Associates on September 28, 2003. Autopsy was performed at Rapella Memorial Hospital morgue. Whether Dr. Guru Singh is board certified in forensic pathology or whether he is certified in anatomic or clinical pathology is not known. The blood sample was drawn from the chest cavity during autopsy. Despite the multiple traumas involved, Dr. Singh did not collect vitreous fluid for alcohol analysis. He did not make an effort to determine the time of death.

There were superficial bruises of the head and neck with no fractures. Two liters of blood were collected from the left cavity of the chest by compressing the left lung. Less than 50 ml of blood was present in the peritoneal cavity. There were limb injuries, a massive hemothorax in the left chest cavity (2 L of blood), and 100 ml of blood in the right chest cavity. The stomach contained 40 ml of a thick, brown, mucous fluid. At autopsy, blood, urine, and brain tissue were collected and sent to Chadda's Biochemistry, Inc. The results showed 0.17% of blood ethanol, and 0.22% of urine ethanol. No vitreous fluid was collected and analyzed. The stomach contents were not analyzed. Total amount of urine present in the urinary bladder was not documented. The methods used for ethanol analysis are not given.

According to the accepted practices of forensic pathology, ideally two blood specimens need to be collected from two different sites (17). In addition to blood, vitreous humor and stomach contents should be collected in all postmortem cases (2). This is important in view of the fact that the deceased suffered massive trauma and the alcohol present in the stomach could contaminate the blood in the chest cavity (17). Although urine is an excellent specimen for drug screening, no direct relationship exists between urine concentration of ethanol and degree of impairment. Urine alcohol cannot be extrapolated to BAC. Again, analysis of alcohol in brain tissue is useful to indicate that the deceased was exposed to alcohol. There are no studies in scientific literature to correlate brain alcohol levels with impairment. Specimens other than whole blood can be of some diagnostic help, but it must be clearly understood that they cannot reliably be converted by an equivalent "average" factor to get BAC (18-23).

21.2.5   Blood Alcohol Concentration

BAC depends on several factors as stated earlier (21). In a normal healthy male weighing 200 pounds, one alcoholic drink is expected to give a BAC of 0.02% (24). Mr. Derry weighed 230 pounds and one alcoholic drink was expected to give a BAC of 0.17%. Alcohol from blood dissipates at the rate of 0.02% per hour (25).

According to forensic pathology and toxicology experts, when traumatic injury occurs and if unabsorbed ethanol is present in the stomach, contamination of transthoracic blood samples can artificially elevate BAC (26). In such cases, it is recommended that heart blood samples from the intact heart and vitreous fluid from the eye be analyzed to rule out contamination with stomach alcohol. Frequently, a blood sample obtained by transthoracic needle aspiration or cardiac puncture may give a falsely elevated BAC. This is due to permeation of alcohol from the GI tract to the thoracic cavity (10). It is important that the BAC is representative of the circulatory alcohol. The alcohol contained in the intact vascular system is the indicator of the pharmacologic effects of ethanol. Therefore, it is vital for proper interpretation of BAC that the blood sample obtained be valid. Urine alcohol is not useful in predicting BAC. All that urine alcohol concentration reflects is an average over the period of time the urine was produced. By virtue of this, urine concentrations are not useful for predicting blood alcohol (19-23).

21.2.6   Presumptive Impairment of Mr. Donard
Derry's Driving Abilities

Mr. Derry's job took him to several places of entertainment and nightclubs. As a director of sales for the Xyz TV station, he often went to clubs for promotional events. He arrived at Erra Matti club at 1:00 a.m. and left at approximately 3:45 a.m. He was seen driving on the road at 4:00 a.m.

No evidence has been available about the number of drinks Mr. Derry had throughout the evening starting at 8:00 p.m. According to Marcy Malman, they visited Surya's and other nightclubs starting at 8:00 p.m. Mr. Derry went to these places with his co-workers. Marcy Malman says that they walked together to Mr. Derry's car at approximately 12:30 a.m. Marcy Malman says that Mr. Derry did not appear intoxicated. When he entered Erra Matti's at 1:00 a.m., there was a time lapse of 5 hours from the time he entered Kona Seema's. A normal healthy male is expected to dissipate 0.02% alcohol per hour from blood. Therefore, in these five hours he must have dissipated at least 0.1% alcohol from blood. In other words, he was sober and other witnesses corroborated this.

At 4:00 a.m., he appeared sober according to an eyewitness account. The accident happened at 5:05 a.m. There was a time lapse of approximately 90 minutes between the time he left Erra Matti's and the accident. Therefore, he was expected still to be absorbing alcohol from the GI tract. Indeed, there was fluid in his stomach, which if analyzed could have confirmed the presence of alcohol. This alcohol was in the process of absorption and permeating further into his bloodstream, body fluids, and tissues until the time he was declared dead at 8:21 a.m. There was a time lapse of nearly 2 hours from the time he left Erra Matti's to the time of his accident. Assuming he died instantly and 0.17% BAC determined on the blood drawn at autopsy was the BAC at the time of accident, then one has to add 0.04%, the alcohol he was expected to dissipate from blood in 2 hours. Then his total BAC would come to 0.21% at the time of the accident. To get a BAC of 0.21% Mr. Derry should have consumed at least 12 to 13 drinks in a short span of 2 hours at Erra Matti's. This is unlikely and underscores the contention that Mr. Derry's BAC determined from the blood drawn at autopsy was contaminated with the unabsorbed alcohol in the stomach. The sanctity of the samples and the conditions of their storage between October 2 and October 3 in the laboratory is not known. Whether the laboratory has restricted access to the storage area where the samples were held is also not known. The method used in alcohol determination is not known. If they used an enzymatic method of alcohol dehydrogenase, then the alcohol result would also be falsely elevated in a person with multiple traumas (27).

21.2.7 Conclusions

There is no scientific evidence to show that a 0.17% BAC obtained from autopsy blood was Mr. Derry's BAC at the time of the accident. In fact, the evidence points out that Mr. Derry was not intoxicated at the time of the accident and was not impaired to cause the accident.

It can be concluded with a reasonable degree of medical and scientific certainty that:

1. Mr. Donard Derry was still absorbing alcohol from his GI tract at the time of the accident.
2. Because of massive injuries to his chest and abdomen, the blood drawn at autopsy was contaminated with unabsorbed alcohol from his stomach, which resulted in a falsely elevated BAC.
3. Mr. Derry was not intoxicated at the time of the accident and was not impaired to cause the accident.

21.3   Platinum Salts and Development of Asthma

21.3.1   Legal Aspects: Occupational Asthma

This case is about Mr. Chuck Williams, who developed occupational asthma secondary to his exposure to toxic metals while working at AutoCat plant. He filed a civil lawsuit against his employer for monetary compensation for his pain and suffering, development of occupational asthma resulting in his permanent disability, and loss of gainful employment. Subsequently, he went on workers' compensation.

21.3.2   Medical Aspects: Metal Toxicity

Exposure to complex platinum salts at the workplace is a well-known cause of occupational asthma. There is enough evidence to suggest that other precious metals may also sensitize the workers.

21.3.3   Factual Background

This case is about Chuck Williams, who is an African American male, 48 years of age, 6 feet 1 inch tall and weighing 237 pounds. He was a high school graduate and had 2 years of college education. He started working at AutoCat, Inc. in November 2000. This employer manufactures catalytic converters for several automobiles. The manufacturing process involves impregnation of precious metals including platinum on substrates. This manufacturing facility has several buildings including Levon 2 and Levon 3. Chuck started his work with this employer as a line loader in Levon 2. He continued there for the next 26 months. He also worked in the unit of impregnation of precious metals. His work also involved cleaning out batch tanks and cleaning floors with mops and buffers. The air from the knives blows out wash coat, which would fall onto the floor and under the belts. This dries out to dust and this dust had to be cleaned and swept several times during a shift. The area is filled with the smell of acid and ammonia. Even though Chuck was required to wear protective gear, he was never given a respirator. The ventilation in several areas was poor. Chuck worked 80 to 90 hours per week. Because of the smell of concentrated fumes and the dust, he had difficulty breathing at work. When he complained to his supervisors about his breathing difficulties, he was asked to go out and get some fresh air.

21.3.4   Health Problems of Chuck Williams

Chuck developed weakness, shortness of breath, cough, and chest tightness, and was coughing up black mucus. In the initial stages, these symptoms appeared only at work, and decreased when he was outside the work environment. Later, these symptoms persisted in or outside the work environment. Even though he smoked cigarettes since he was 20 years of age, he never experienced asthma-like symptoms prior to his working at the AutoCat plant. He went to the emergency room of County Memorial Hospital after a severe episode of shortness of breath. During the course of the next few years, several physicians saw him for his persistent symptoms of weakness, shortness of breath, and wheezing. Before his employment at AutoCat, he was not sensitive to cleaning fluids or perfumes, and had never experienced any breathing problems. The physicians diagnosed him with reactive airways dysfunction syndrome (RADS) and occupational asthma. To treat his asthma, the doctors put him on Albuterol and Advair.

AutoCat has a nurse who attends to the health complaints of the employees. The nurse referred Mr. Williams to a doctor who noted that Mr. Williams was wheezing and breathless at work and had dyspnea, which gets better when he is away from the work site. Dr. Steven Wu examined Mr. Williams and diagnosed him with asthma and RADS. He noted that the patient became inactive with intermittent episodes of shortness of breath. He also advised the patient to use Advair and Albuterol. Spirometry and airflow volume curves suggested that the symptoms were consistent with occupational asthma. Dr. Charlie Egom, Dr. Linda Black, and Dr. Bobby Lee also examined Mr. Williams. All of these physicians agreed that Mr. Williams' symptoms were consistent with asthma. Mr. Williams is continuing his treatment with Dr. Bobby Lee, long after he left the employment of AutoCat.

21.3.5   Material Safety Data Sheets

AutoCat uses several chemicals in the manufacturing process. The material safety data sheets (MSDS) were supplied by the employer from their files, which they were given by the manufacturers of the chemicals used in the AutoCat plant. In addition to these MSDS, the toxicity of these chemicals are published in scientific literature (**5,28**). Toxicity of these chemicals is given next.

21.3.5.1 *Tetramine Platinum (II) Chloride*

This compound is a white crystalline solid and is classified as a toxicant. The platinum halogen salts are toxic and sensitizers. It is known that sensitized persons will develop allergy, asthma, and rhinitis. Allergic reaction to platinum salts may include any of the following: itchy red eyes, watering of the eyes, sneezing, runny nose, chest tightness, wheezing, breathlessness, cough, etc. Exposure to platinum salts in exceedingly small amounts even below the level of chemical detection will produce symptoms in sensitized persons. Continued exposure will give symptoms of increasing severity and can eventually lead to chronic asthma. There is a risk of anaphylactic shock occurring in sensitized persons re-encountering platinum salts. Therefore, if sensitization has developed, further exposure to platinum compounds must not be permitted. It is recommended that workers should wear respirators and fully protective impervious suits.

21.3.5.2 *Tetramine Platinum (II)*

It is recommended that workers should wear protective equipment. Sensitization is possible through skin contact. This platinum compound causes severe allergic reaction, irritation, sensitization reactions, and asthma. Effects include sneezing, coughing, tightness in the chest, dyspnea, and wheezing. Chronic exposure may result in pulmonary fibrosis. Small doses of nitrates may cause weakness, general depression, and headache.

21.3.5.3 *Rhodium (III) Nitrate*

This is a harmful compound. It is a crystalline and yellow-brown in color. Use of a suitable respirator is recommended when high concentrations are present. It is an irritant to the skin and mucous membranes. Sensitization is possible through inhalation. Chronic toxicity includes respiratory irritation and respiratory sensitization.

21.3.5.4 *Palladium (II) Nitrate*

Wearing protective equipment such as a suitable respirator is required when high concentrations are present. No sensitizing effects are known. The acute and chronic toxicity of this compound in humans is not fully understood.

21.3.5.5 *Nickel (II) Oxide*

This chemical may cause cancer by irritation. It may cause sensitization by skin contact. Chronic exposure may cause a form of dermatitis called nickel itch, and may cause intestinal disorders and convulsions. This compound is classified as a carcinogen.

21.3.5.6 *Aluminum Oxide*

This white odorless compound may cause gastric and intestinal disorders, coughing, and breathing difficulty. This compound is also implicated in Alzheimer's disease. Inhalation of aluminum-containing dust may cause pulmonary disease.

21.3.5.7 *Barium Sulfate*

Hazard description is not available. Use of a suitable respirator is recommended when high concentrations are present. Sensitizing effects are known.

21.3.5.8 *Neodymium Oxide*

This product is a hygroscopic lump that is odorless and light blue in color. No sensitizing affects are known.

21.3.5.9 *Cerium Zirconium Oxide*

Cerium salts increase blood coagulation rate. The acute and chronic toxicity of this substance is not fully known.

21.3.5.10 *Ammonium Hydroxide*

This is a colorless liquid compound with strong ammonia smell. Inhalation may result in respiratory effects such as inflammation, wheezing, edema, chemical pneumonitis, shortness of breath, headache, nausea, and vomiting.

21.3.5.11 *Ammonium Nitrate*

This is a crystalline solid.

21.3.5.12 *Nitric Acid*

This highly corrosive liquid burns the skin and other areas upon contact. Inhalation of vapors or mist can cause burns in the respiratory tract resulting in lung injury.

21.3.5.13 *Nitrosol (Hydroxyethyl Cellulose)*

This is a powder, white to tan in color, and is odorless. This is not classified as a major toxicant.

21.3.6 Occupational Asthma

Occupational asthma is characterized by variable airflow limitation and airway hyper-responsiveness due to causes and conditions attributable to a particular occupational environment and not to stimuli encountered outside the workplace. There is agreement that the syndrome of chest tightness, wheezing, and shortness of breath appear after a latent period of occupational exposure. A variety of chemicals and agents of biological origin have been described as causes of occupational asthma (**29,30**). In the present case, based on the MSDS supplied by AutoCat, the evidence from scientific literature (**5,28**), and the working conditions as reported by Chuck, it can be concluded that Chuck was exposed to various precious metal salts including platinum during the production process of catalysts for cars.

Occupational exposure to complex platinum salts is a well-known cause of occupational asthma. This conclusion is based on studies of platinum refinery workers and workers in platinum catalyst plants. There is also evidence to suggest that other precious metals such as palladium (Pd) or rhodium (Rh) may also sensitize workers.

The metals of the platinum family include ruthenium (Rn), rhodium (Rh), palladium (pd), osmium (Os), iridium (Ir), and platinum (Pt). These rare metals are often collectively called precious metals. These metals are used for various applications from jewelry to catalysts, electron microscopy, and various high technology sectors including the metallization of electronic parts (**30,31**).

Of all these precious metals, only platinum is known to be a cause of occupational asthma. The strong sensitization potential of complex platinum salts has been well documented. It is concluded that both nonspecific and specific bronchial responsiveness do not decrease in individuals with asthma caused by platinum salts after removal from exposure. In one study reported in the literature, they examined workers in a catalyst production plant and concluded that asthma and rhinitis are caused by exposure to platinum salts. It is well established from studies reported in scientific and medical literature involving platinum refinery workers and catalyst plant workers that exposure to platinum salts has the potential to cause asthma and rhinitis. The symptoms were associated with the degree of exposure. It is known from the literature that asymptomatic subjects sensitized to platinum salts will invariably develop allergic symptoms if not transferred to places without exposure (**32,33**). Even though smoking is a risk factor for platinum salt sensitization, the degree of exposure and duration of exposure to platinum salts will definitely lead to the development of occupational asthma (**30**). Once symptoms are detected, workers should be removed from high exposure areas. Otherwise, the workers will develop serious occupational asthma.

21.3.7   Work Environment at AutoCat Plant

Based on the deposition statement of Mr. Chuck Williams and the sequence of events leading to his development of occupational asthma at AutoCat plant, one can conclude that the plant is being operated with less stringent controls to hazard exposure. There are no adequate safety controls to ensure worker health and well-being. One nurse works as a clearinghouse to refer workers to a doctor if they have health problems. Apparently, the nurse is not up-to-date and knowledgeable of occupational health literature and may not be aware of the results reported in scientific and medical literature that platinum salts cause occupational asthma. The most hazardous area in the catalyst plant is the impregnation of the devices by platinum salts (33). In other catalyst plants in the world, this process is performed entirely by robots. In this plant, the workers manually add platinum salts to batches.

There are no data available regarding periodic analysis of air quality of the plant with respect to particulate content and chemical composition. Whether OSHA did periodic inspections of the plant is not known. The plant does not provide respirators to workers in the plant to minimize the inhalation and exposure to platinum salts. The conditions as reported in Levon 2 and Levon 3 by Mr. Williams are less than ideal for worker safety and health. There are no periodic medical examinations of the workers, which should include analysis of blood and urine for platinum levels. The plant has no periodic medical surveillance programs. It is well established that medical surveillance can prevent the development of occupational asthma caused by platinum salt exposure. It is also well established that symptoms of occupational asthma persist in a high percentage of subjects after allergen exposure. The symptoms get worse if the workers showing these symptoms are not removed from the areas of high exposure. Medical surveillance programs are important to prevent onset of health problems and to remove the workers from the work area causing the health problems in the initial reversible phase (34,35).

The strong sensitization potential of complex platinum salts has been well documented in numerous studies on workers from precious metal refineries. Sensitization is generally considered to occur through hypersensitivity reaction mediated by immunoglobulin E (IgE). This explains why skin prick testing is used for detection of platinum salt exposure and also for the assessment of clinical diagnosis of occupational asthma (30,36). AutoCat performed no such medical surveillance or skin prick tests for the detection of serum or urine platinum. AutoCat did not conduct skin prick tests for employees when skin prick tests have 100% positive predictive value for symptoms and signs of platinum salt sensitivity. It is unfortunate that several doctors including allergists and pulmonologists treating Mr. Williams never conducted skin prick tests or ordered serum and urine screens for analysis. The only thing they did was order lung function tests, diagnosed asthma, and medically managed the patient with Albuterol and Advair.

Unhealthy work conditions at the AutoCat plant and the lack of programs for workers' health and well-being are unfortunate. The lack of medical surveillance and periodic tests for the assessment of platinum salt exposure contributed to the development of occupational asthma of Mr. Williams.

21.3.8   Conclusions

Based on published medical and scientific literature, it can be concluded with a reasonable degree of scientific certainty that:

1. AutoCat maintained unhealthy work conditions in its catalyst plant.
2. Workers are exposed to various chemicals and precious metal salts, particularly to toxic levels of platinum salts.
3. They have no established program in place for periodic medical surveillance of workers. Exposure levels to platinum were never tested by skin prick tests and platinum levels in blood and urine were never determined.
4. Chuck Williams was exposed to toxic levels of platinum and developed serious health consequences resulting in asthma.

21.4   Toxicity of Deicer Mist

21.4.1   Legal Aspects: Deicer Fumes and Accidental Fractures

This case is about Mr. Bill Brown, a truck driver, who was working for Three Rivers Transport. On the day of the accident, he took a truck filled with deicer and pumped it into a mine. The deicer was leaking from the pipes, so he got under the truck to stop the leak. He lost consciousness, and his left arm got caught up in the pumping machinery resulting in multiple fractures. He contends that he cannot work and is on disability. He is demanding monthly income and other benefits under workers' compensation,

21.4.2   Medical Aspects: Toxicity of Diethylene Glycol

Mr. Bill Brown was exposed to mist of the deicer SRA-7000, which contained diethylene glycol. Diethylene glycol is similar to ethylene glycol in toxicity and causes CNS depression, drowsiness, coma, and finally death. Mr. Brown lost consciousness and his left arm was caught up in the machinery resulting in multiple fractures.

21.4.3   Factual Background

Bill Brown is a Caucasian male, 50 years of age, who was involved in a serious accident on November 22, 2004. This accident caused a fracture of his left hand. Mr. Brown is a tanker truck driver, who was pumping liquid deicer from his truck into a mine. While trying to stop a leak from the hose around the packing gland, he got under the truck and was exposed to the mist of the liquid deicer and lost consciousness. His left arm was caught up in the machinery resulting in an open fracture of his left arm. A helicopter took him to Villanova Medical Center. He was admitted on November 22, 2004 and discharged three weeks later. After a series of surgical procedures, he is still under physiotherapy. The details of the incident are as follows.

Mr. Brown is 6 feet 2 inches tall and weighed 170 pounds on the day of the accident. Mr. Brown was in the Army and retired after 20 years. He worked as a boiler operator and is knowledgeable about several types of machinery. He moved to Nevada after retirement and started working as a truck driver, driving a freightliner. He has worked for Three Rivers Transportation since January 2002 as a truck driver and has hauled loads as required by the company. He received a hard hat, face shield, goggles, and an acid suit. He received monthly training from his terminal manager.

On the day of the accident, Mr. Brown left home, drove to Jenova, and got his truck and everything needed to transport the deicer. He went to the plant at Plano at 7:00 am. His truck was loaded with deicer SRA-7000 and he drove to the mine where it was to be delivered. He hooked up the air system in his truck and pressurized the tank. He hooked up the hoses and made sure everything was in order. He started unloading the liquid from the truck, sat outside the truck, and was watching the liquid deicer being pumped. He went around the truck and noticed that it was leaking around the packing gland. He adjusted the packing gland to stop the leak. Apparently, the leak happened two more times. He went underneath the truck to stop the leak and while doing this he was exposed to the mist that was coming out of the leak. He became unconscious and he thinks that his left hand was caught up and entangled in the PTO shaft. His injuries included a large cut on his back and a compound fracture in the left arm.

21.4.4 Hospital Course

Mr. Brown was admitted to the Villanova Medical Center Emergency Department. He was given multiple pain medications with IV drips. He underwent several surgical procedures and was discharged. Analysis of blood, urine, and other body fluids was unremarkable and his labs were mostly normal. There was no ethanol in serum. His urine was analyzed for drugs of abuse on the same day of admission. The drug labs were all negative suggesting that Mr. Brown was not intoxicated due to drugs of abuse.

21.4.5 Composition of Liquid Deicer, SRA-7000

According to MSDS supplied by the company, the liquid being hauled in the truck was SRA-7000. This is a blend of calcium chloride, diethylene glycol, and water. This product was purchased from De Carlo Tetra Performance Chemicals. A sample was removed from the truck and subjected to quality control analysis. SRA-7000 in the truck contained 1126.94 gallons of water, 235.4 gallons of diethylene glycol, and 2842.5 gallons of 35% solution of calcium chloride in water. Inhalation of spray or mist can cause irritation to the nose, throat, and lungs. Even though the material is stated as non-hazardous under normal circumstances, intake of diethylene glycol is known to be toxic and can result in fatalities. Even though he did not ingest it by mouth, inhalation of the mist resulted in rapid absorption through his lungs.

21.4.5.1 Diethylene Glycol

Diethylene glycol is a colorless, odorless, clear liquid. It is miscible with water in any ratio. It has many industrial uses. It is a component of antifreeze, brake fluids, cosmetics, inks, and drying agents, and it is used as a plasticizer. The toxicity of diethylene glycol is similar to ethylene glycol and clearly is a CNS depressant. It has a low inhalation hazard because of its low vapor pressure; however, inhalation of the mist or aerosol is to be avoided. Workplace levels for vapors and aerosols cannot exceed 50 ppm. In case of accidental release of diethylene glycol, use of a full-face positive air pressure respirator is recommended. Even though the toxicokinetics in humans is not completely understood, its toxic nature is confirmed by animal studies. Several human cases were reported in the medical literature. Several children in Haiti died in 1995 and 1996 following the consumption of medication containing diethylene glycol. Similar other cases in children were reported in other countries as well. A 24-year-old man developed encephalopathy and rapidly became quadriplegic following ingestion of a solution containing diethylene glycol (**5,37-44**). Thus, the toxicity of diethylene glycol is well established.

21.4.6 Health Consequences of Bill Brown Subsequent to His Accident

Mr. Brown is a married man with normal health. Before the accident, he was not under the care of a doctor. He drinks beer during the weekends and he had a previous history of smoking for three years. He was never unconscious before the accident and he never experienced dizzy spells. In the Army, he was a boiler technician and acquired the skills to operate several machines. The laboratory analyses of his body fluids at Villanova Medical Center Hospital after the accident revealed that he had no drugs or alcohol in his system. The accident resulted in fractures of his left arm with excruciating pain. At the hospital, he underwent multiple surgical procedures. After discharge from the hospital, he is still undergoing physiotherapy to acquire as much functional use of his left arm as possible. He has not worked after his accident.

21.4.7   Conclusions

It is concluded with a reasonable degree of scientific certainty that:

1. Mr. Brown was alert when he was unloading the deicer from his truck into the mine.
2. Mr. Brown was exposed to the mist of diethylene glycol when he went under the truck and was trying to stop a leak from the hose at the packing gland.
3. He inhaled the diethylene glycol mist, which caused CNS depression and he became unconscious. This resulted in multiple fractures of his left arm when it was caught up in the machinery.
4. Three Rivers Transport was negligent in not providing a respirator with positive air pressure.
5. His employer did not warn Mr. Brown about the toxicity of diethylene glycol; therefore, they are responsible for his accident.

21.5   Death Due to Prescription Medication Overdose

21.5.1   Legal Aspects: Accidental Drug Overdose and Death

This case is about Richard Davis, who died on February 19, 2006. He was 39 years old and his death was ruled accidental due to combined actions of prescription medications, morphine, and OxyContin. His wife, Mrs. Mary Davis, brought a civil suit against Pf United Contractors and alleged that they were responsible for his back injury at work, which made him dependent on prescription pain medications. This ultimately resulted in accidental overdose and death. His employer contends that they are not responsible for his death as he overdosed himself.

21.5.2   Medical Aspects: Combined Toxicity of Morphine and OxyContin

Mr. Davis died due to accidental overdose of pain medications. Autopsy revealed high levels of morphine and oxycodone in his blood. Combined toxicity of these two drugs resulted in his death.

21.5.3   Factual Background

Mr. Davis was with his wife Mary Davis at their home in Fishkill, NY. His death was ruled accidental by the coroner and was caused by the combined actions of morphine and oxycodone.

Mr. Davis worked as a construction laborer for Pf United 1 Contractors. On July 22, 2000, he injured his back when he was working with a jackhammer. Subsequent to this injury, he was in constant pain and had to go on total disability. He was under the care of several physicians and underwent several procedures to relieve his back pain. None of these procedures helped him alleviate his pain. As a part of his treatment, he was put on 90 mg of MS Contin, three times a day, and Endocet, two times a day by Dr. Robert Gartelli, a pain specialist. Dr. Gartelli testified that Mr. Davis signed a contract not to doctor shop and obtain these prescriptions from any other source. Dr. Gartelli further stated that he had no indication that Mr. Davis was doctor shopping or obtaining these medications through other pharmacies.

Mr. Davis had no MS Contin or Endocet for nearly two weeks and obtained prescriptions from Dr. Gartelli. Mr. Davis and his wife had his prescriptions filled at Rex Pharmacy on February 18, 2006 at 4:30 p.m. His wife told the police that she was with her husband the whole day. According to Duchess County Prosecutor's Office Supplemental Report, Mrs. Davis told the police that after they got the prescription filled by the pharmacy, she thought that her husband took twice the prescribed dose on a bench in front of the pharmacy. She testified to the judge at trial that she was not sure of her husband taking the double dose. Later they went shopping in the mall and had pizza. She further testified that they were together the whole day. They drove back to their house. On their way home, Mr. Davis left the medicine bottles in the glove compartment of their car. She is sure that her husband did not take any other doses.

Mrs. Davis told police that after they went home, her husband complained that he was tired and his legs were numb. She helped him to bed around midnight. They slept in the same bed. She woke up at 7:00 a.m. and thought her husband was sleeping. She went back to the bedroom to wake her husband at approximately 11:30 a.m. and found him unresponsive. She then called 911.

The police arrived at 11:41 a.m. and found that Richard was dead. There was no evidence of external trauma. The police found that the victim's arms were in full rigor mortis. The officer accompanied Mrs. Davis to her car to retrieve the medicine bottles from the glove compartment.

21.5.4 Autopsy

Mr. Davis's body was moved to Underwood Hospital Morgue where Dr. Leela Sunderan performed the autopsy on February 20, 2006. The manner of death was ruled accidental and the cause of death was determined to be combined toxicity of morphine and oxycodone. There was no external trauma. The rest of the autopsy findings were unremarkable. The stomach contained approximately 300 ml of a thick tan liquid with fragments of food. Histology was not done. Specimens submitted for toxicology analysis included blood, brain, and liver. Stomach contents were not submitted for toxicology analysis as the coroner ruled the cause of death accidental and she did not believe that Mr. Davis intentionally ingested a large quantity of pills. Toxicology did not detect ethanol or any other drugs of abuse in his blood. Morphine was 81 mg/L (therapeutic range, 0.01 to 0.10 mg/L and oxycodone was 0.78 mg/L (therapeutic range is 0.01 to 0.06 mg/L).

21.5.5 Presumptive Dose Ingested

Based on the drug levels in his autopsy blood, it is possible to calculate the amount of prescription drugs Mr. Davis ingested after he had the prescription filled by Rex Pharmacy. He was given MS Contin, which is a slow-release morphine sulfate. The prescription was filled as 60- and 30-mg tablets and he was asked to take 90 mg every 8 hours. He was also given Endocet tablets, which have 7.5 mg of oxycodone and 325 mg of acetaminophen. He was asked to take one tablet every 12 hours.

Using volume of distribution (Vd) (L/kg), it is possible to calculate the dose ingested (D) provided the body weight (B.wt) in kilograms and the drug concentration (C) in mg/liter in blood are known (17,45,46).

$$D = B.wt \times Vd \times C$$

(Vd for morphine is 2 to 5 L/kg)
(Vd for oxycodone is 1.8 to 3.7 L/kg)

Mr. Davis weighed 180 pounds, or 82 kg. Average Vd for morphine is 3.5 L/kg. The average Vd for oxycodone is 2.8 L/kg.

21.5.5.1 Morphine Ingested

Blood levels of morphine were 0.81 mg/L.

$$D = 82 \times 3.5 \times 0.81$$
$$= 232 \text{ mg}$$

Therefore, Mr. Davis ingested four tablets of 60-mg MS Contin.

21.5.5.2 Oxycodone Ingested

Blood levels of oxycodone were 0.078 mg/L.

$$D = 82 \times 2.8 \times 0.078 = 17.9 \text{ mg}$$

Therefore, Mr. Davis took two tablets of Endocet.

21.5.6 Toxicity of MS Contin and Endocet

There is no evidence to suggest that Mr. Davis intentionally overdosed himself. The police officer noticed that Mr. Davis's arms were in full rigor mortis. Rigor mortis usually develops 6 to 12 hours after death (**3**). Richard and Mary went to bed around midnight. The police arrived at the scene at 11:41 a.m. Therefore, the death must have occurred a few hours after Richard and Mary went to bed. The medicine bottles were in the glove compartment of the car. She retrieved them for police. This underscores the fact that death was accidental due to ingestion of two doses of these medications at one time.

MS Contin is a controlled-release tablet containing morphine sulfate and is prescribed for the treatment of pain. Morphine is an opioid drug extracted from opium. While regular morphine is rapidly absorbed and is given every four hours, MS Contin is a controlled-release tablet and is taken every 8 to 12 hours depending upon patients' needs. It is clearly stated on the prescription that the patient has to swallow it. If the tablet is chewed or crushed, a dangerously large amount of morphine could enter the blood stream at once resulting in a fatal outcome. If for some reason a dose is missed, the patient is asked to wait until it is time to take the next dose. The patient is always warned not to take two doses together as this will result in toxic levels of morphine in the blood. Doses greater than 30 mg parenteral and 100 mg orally are toxic to non-tolerant adults. In fact, death may occur following doses of 120 mg or more (**2**). Endocet contains oxycodone and acetaminophen. Oxycodone is a semi-synthetic narcotic used in the treatment of pain. Richard was asked to take one tablet every 12 hours.

21.5.7 Conclusions

Based on the available evidence, it can be concluded with a reasonable degree of scientific and medical certainty that:

1. Mr. Davis died because of combined acute intoxication of morphine and oxycodone.
2. Death was accidental; Mr. Davis was ignorant that two doses of morphine and oxycodone taken together would result in a fatal outcome.
3. Even though he was injured at work, his death was due to his own carelessness.

21.6 Sodium Bichromate Exposure and Development of Non-Hodgkin's Lymphoma

21.6.1 Legal Aspects: Sodium Bichromate and Non-Hodgkin's Lymphoma

This case is about Mr. Darryl Wells, who developed non-Hodgkin's lymphoma. Mr. Wells attributed this to his exposure to sodium bichromate at

Greenland Tube Company. Mr. Wells succumbed to complications of the disease and died a few months later. His wife sued the Greenland Tube Company for monetary compensation for loss of her husband's employment, his pain, suffering, and finally his death.

21.6.2   Medical Aspects: Chromium Toxicity

Chromium is an established human and animal carcinogen. Mr. Wells was exposed to sodium bichromate and other carcinogens at his workplace, which resulted in the development of non-Hodgkin's lymphoma.

21.6.3   Factual Background

Mr. Wells lived in Mars, Pennsylvania. He was a 47-year-old African American male, 6 feet 2 inches tall and weighing approximately 245 pounds. He worked for Greenland Tube Company until April 12, 2006. Actually, he started working at AK Steel in 2000, and Greenland Tube Company acquired this tube manufacturing plant in April 2002. He was working as a maintenance millwright. He was responsible for routine maintenance and repairs of all the machinery in the plant whenever needed.

The last day he worked at the plant was on April 12, 2006. He developed pain below his rib cage and his family physician sent him for further tests. His CT scan and other studies revealed the presence of a 16 × 8 cm mesenteric mass. He was hospitalized for two days for biopsy of the mass and the pathologist identified it as malignant follicular lymphoma. Dr. Theresa Lob is a clinician affiliated with United Medical Hospital and was treating Mr. Wells. This follicular lymphoma is also called non-Hodgkin's lymphoma. Mr. Wells was put on chemotherapy and was made to wear a narcotic patch for pain control. Non-Hodgkin's lymphoma is an aggressive tumor and cannot be surgically resected.

21.6.4   Social and Work History

Mr. Wells was married and lived with his wife. Although he smoked as a teenager, he did not currently smoke. His earlier health history includes contact dermatitis, which can be attributed to his exposure to methyl ethyl ketone. Before 2000, he worked for nearly 15 years at Baja Industries at Johannesburg, Pennsylvania. During long layoffs at this company, he also worked at Mord Corporation, Erie, Pennsylvania in their mailroom. Before 1985, he worked as a laborer, overhead crane man, maintenance mechanic, and area millwright.

21.6.5 Brief Details of Pipe Manufacturing at Greenland Tube Company

Greenland Tube Company manufactures steel pipes, which are galvanized by zinc coating. The steel pipes as they come out are dipped into molten zinc. This process occurs in a big tub. The tubes come out of this tub by conveyor belts and are then dipped into a big tub of sodium bichromate. There are protective flashers, but still the solution of this hexavalent chromium salt spills out and the surrounding area is filled with vapors of this solution. As a millwright, when the equipment broke down Mr. Wells had to crawl into the big tub that contained sodium bichromate. The exposure to this chromium salt is quite significant. Cleaning and maintenance of this equipment containing the sodium bichromate is done whenever necessary and the physical exposure to the chemical occurs at least once weekly.

The metal finishing industry uses hexavalent chromium salt for passivation of zinc and aluminum. Zinc is used as a protective coating on mild steel. Zinc coating has valuable characteristics for metal finishing. Zinc coating has the property of self-healing over small scratches. Zinc coating may oxidize. To prevent this oxidation, a passivation process is used. To do this, zinc-coated pipes are dipped in a sodium bichromate solution (**47**).

21.6.6 Lymphomas

Development of malignant tumors does not occur as a single event. It is recognized by scientists in the field of carcinogenesis that tumor development is a multistage process. A normal cell is initiated by exposure to a carcinogen, and this initiated cell remains latent. Subsequent events such as repeated exposure to the same chemical or other chemicals or hormones result in clonal expansion of this initiated cell. This is called promotion. The final stage is progression to a malignant tumor by rapid division of these cancer cells (**48**).

There are two types of lymphomas: Hodgkin's disease and non-Hodgkin's disease. Hodgkin's disease starts in lymphatic tissue, which includes lymph nodes. Because lymphatic tissue is present in many parts of the body, lymphoma can develop almost anywhere. However, it rarely migrates to other parts of the body and is treatable. Non-Hodgkin's lymphoma is many types. They begin with the initiation of a B cell or a T cell. If the cell is exposed to a carcinogen such as sodium bichromate, it becomes a cancer cell. This cancer cell rapidly divides and becomes a tumor, which may metastasize. This cancer is rarely treatable. In the United States, non-Hodgkin's lymphomas are more common than Hodgkin's disease. Non-Hodgkin's lymphomas in the United States are the sixth most common cancer among males and the fifth most common cancer among females (**49-51**).

21.6.7   Carcinogenicity of Chromium

It is established that chromium is an essential trace element for humans and must be supplied in the diet. Deficiency of chromium causes abnormalities in glucose metabolism and insulin function. In spite of its essentiality, chromium is recognized as a human and animal carcinogen (52). Even though it is known that this element causes bronchial, nasal, and lung cancers, it may cause cancers at other sites as well. Modern day chromium exposure occurs from an occupational setting. This includes workers involved in welding, metal grinding, and the leather industry. Mostly hexavalent chromium salts are recognized as human and animal carcinogens. MSDS states that sodium bichromate can enter humans through inhalation, ingestion, and skin contact. Sodium bichromate is a bright orange crystal, classified as a Group 1 carcinogen by IARC, and a recognized carcinogen by NTP. Hexavalent chromium causes cancer in humans and animals and causes genetic toxicity to human and animal cells (53). All industries should control the exposure levels of hexavalent chromium salts for their workers (54,55).

Experimental studies involving guinea pigs show that potassium dichromate sensitization of the animals and subsequent repeated antigenic percutaneous injections over a period of several days caused lymphomas (56). Epidemiological studies showed that two patients exposed to excessive hexavalent chromium salts developed Hodgkin's disease (57). In the United States, non-Hodgkin's lymphomas are lower among African Americans even though their overall cancer incidence is approximately 24% higher than Caucasians. Significant increase in Hodgkin's disease and non-Hodgkin's lymphoma are higher in Caucasian firefighters than African American firefighters. Therefore, the racial predisposition playing a major role in the development of this cancer is ruled out in this case (58).

In fact, the overall exposure levels to sodium bichromate play a major role in the development of non-Hodgkin's lymphoma. One study confirmed the development of more non-Hodgkin's lymphoma among African Americans than among Caucasian workers due to exposure to sodium bichromate in the workplace. This disproportionate increase in non-Hodgkin's lymphoma in this group can be linked directly to the disproportionate exposure of African Americans to hexavalent chromium salts due to their work pattern and job duties. Forty-one percent of African Americans were found to have been assigned to jobs involving exposure to the highest levels of chromate when compared to 16% of Caucasians (59). In any case, this clearly establishes that in addition to lung cancers, sodium bichromate causes non-Hodgkin's lymphoma (52,60).

21.6.8   Conclusions

It can be concluded with a reasonable degree of scientific certainty that:

1. Mr. Wells was exposed to sodium bichromate at the workplace.
2. Sodium bichromate is a human and animal carcinogen and caused his non-Hodgkin's lymphoma.
3. Besides loss of employment, Mr. Wells underwent pain and suffering and this tumor finally killed him.

21.7   Exposure to Carcinogens and Brain Cancer

21.7.1   Legal Aspects: Carcinogen Exposure and Astrocytoma

This case is about Mr. Erick Delmick, who died of astrocytoma. His wife contends that her husband's astrocytoma was caused by his exposure to carcinogens at Bloomfield Power Station where he worked for 30 years. She sued the power plant for monetary compensation for his pain and suffering and loss of income due to his death.

21.7.2   Medical Aspects: Carcinogen-Induced Astrocytoma

Mr. Delmick was exposed to benzene, hydrocarbons, coal dust and fly ash, lead, cadmium, mercury, arsenic, asbestos, and electromagnetic fields (EMFs). Most of these are established or suspected animal and human carcinogens. This exposure to carcinogens resulted in the development of brain cancer (**61**).

21.7.3   Factual Background

Mr. Delmick was a 56-year-old Caucasian male, who worked as an outage coordinator and died on July 12, 2002 due to astrocytoma. He was hired as a repair-helper in 1970 at Bloomfield Power Station. He was promoted to shift maintenance supervisor in 1975. After 15 years, he was promoted to outage coordinator and worked in that position until his death in July 2002.

During his work at the power plant, Mr. Delmick was exposed to high EMFs. In addition, during the first 15 years of his employment as a repair-helper he used large quantities of degreasers. These degreasers were used on a daily basis. He used Varsol initially and later the company replaced it with benzene-free Varsol. He also used Electrosol and several other aromatic hydrocarbon degreasers. To repair the equipment, he had to separate the parts and degrease the equipment. The parts and motors were put in a tank containing Varsol. If the equipment or the parts were large, he used to spray them with degreasers under pressure. The sprayed Varsol got into the air and he was exposed to this spray. There was no ventilation in the plant where the repairs were done. There was no protective equipment. The original Varsol was used up until mid-1980. This Varsol contained as much as 25% benzene. Management removed this Varsol tank from the plant as a hazardous waste. Later on, the original Varsol was replaced with benzene-free Varsol. Besides Varsol, Mr. Delmick used several other degreasers as sprays, which contained aromatic hydrocarbons. He also used Electrosol as a degreaser, which contained trichloroethane.

In addition, a Varsol tank was used by all the workers as the primary wash station and they put their hands into the tank to remove the grease off their hands. After the grease was out, they went to a sink and washed their hands again. The work area had fly ash floating around all over. Fly ash contains heavy metals such as mercury, arsenic, and lead. He was also exposed to asbestos. In addition, Mr. Delmick was exposed to EMFs. He and the other workers were not provided with MSDS for various chemicals that might be present in the workplace.

21.7.4 Medical History

Mr. Delmick was married and lived with his wife at home. His past medical history included Type 1 diabetes for which he took insulin. He had kidney disease, hypertension, peripheral neuropathy, and proliferative retinopathy. He was a smoker earlier but he quit smoking a few years ago. His physician's notes indicate that in early April 2002, he was agitated and confused. On April 30, 2002, he was seen in the emergency room at Judy Memorial Hospital. He complained of shortness of breath, increased right-side weakness, and deterioration in the level of his consciousness. He was transferred to Eastern Spokane University Hospital at Bethany. The CT scan showed chest pulmonary embolus. The CT scan of the brain detected a low-grade glioma. Further pathology examination confirmed the presence of diffuse astrocytoma, Grade II. It was not possible to surgically remove the tumor. He died on June 11, 2002. The cause of death was due to astrocytoma.

21.7.5 Astrocytomas

Astrocytomas are brain tumors that belong to a general class of gliomas. Gliomas can be benign or malignant. The astrocytomas are most common in adults, primarily in middle-aged men. Astrocytomas originate from astrocytes. The latent period is quite long. The astrocytomas are malignant and cannot be removed surgically. Astrocytomas of any type and at any age are infiltrative tumors that act as mass lesions wherever they are found. They cause symptoms related to the area in which they are found. Astrocytomas make up 60% of brain tumors. Grade II astrocytomas are seen in cerebral hemispheres of 20- to 40-year-old individuals and high grade astrocytomas, which are most malignant in their course, are seen in patients in their 50s and 60s. Etiologies of brain cancers include exposure to radiation, chemicals, pesticides, polycyclic aromatic hydrocarbons, and nitroso compounds as well as chlorinated hydrocarbons (**62**).

21.7.6 Toxicity of Chemicals, Heavy Metals, and EMF Present at the Power Plant

21.7.6.1 *Benzene*

Benzene is a highly flammable organic solvent with a sweet aromatic smell. The content of benzene in gasoline varies between 1.5 and 6%. Benzene is a product of petroleum refining. It is commercially prepared from petroleum naphtha and purified by washing with water. Chronic exposure leads to leukemia. Early symptoms of exposure to benzene include fatigue, headache, weakness, and bleeding gums. Anemia and bleeding disorders can occur (**5**).

Exposure to hydrocarbons generated at the petroleum factory can occur through inhalation of vapors or through dermal contact. Of special concern is benzene, which has been linked to an increased risk of leukemia (**63**). For nearly 100 years, the acute and chronic toxicity of benzene has been well documented by clinicians, epidemiologists, and occupational safety experts. Benzene is known to suppress the production of red and white blood cells and decrease cells in the bone marrow. As early as 1930, red and white cell counts were monitored for managing employee risk. Particularly meaningful is the finding by several researchers regarding the progression of aplastic anemia in benzene-exposed individuals through a pre-leukemia phase into frank acute leukemia. Benzene was declared a human carcinogen. This chemical was known to cause other cancers in other sites as well. There are numerous case reports of long delays between the cessation of known benzene exposure and the onset of leukemia. It may have a latency of 20 to 30 years after exposure to benzene (**64**). Benzene toxicity to humans exposed at the workplace is characterized by early reversible hemato-toxicity or irreversible bone marrow damage with prolonged exposure to high doses (**65**).

As stated previously, benzene can cause cancers in other sites, besides leukemia and lymphomas. National Toxicology Program (NTP), Toxicology and Carcinogenesis group conducted animal studies in 1986. These studies showed that in male rats benzene caused zymbal gland carcinomas, squamous cell papillomas, and squamous cell carcinomas of the oral cavity. In addition, benzene caused squamous cell papillomas and squamous cell carcinomas of the skin. Similar results were seen in female rats as well. In male mice, benzene caused zymbal gland squamous cell carcinomas, malignant lymphomas, alveolar and bronchiolar carcinomas, and squamous cell carcinomas of the perputial gland. In female mice, benzene increased the incidence of malignant lymphomas, ovarian granulosa cell tumors, ovarian benign mixed tumors, carcinomas and arcinor sarcomas, and zymbal gland squamous cell tumors (5). A Canadian study investigated benzene exposure in the occupational setting and concluded that benzene caused increased incidence of brain cancer and mortality in workers due to occupational exposure (66).

21.7.6.2 Hydrocarbons
Benzene-free Varsol contains several hydrocarbons produced from petroleum distillate. These hydrocarbons, when inhaled, can produce transient CNS depression, pulmonary damage, hypoxia, cardiac problems, and finally death. This includes many chlorinated and aromatic hydrocarbons. Chronic exposure can produce a variety of cancers. Excess deaths from bone, brain, and bladder cancer attributed to exposure of these chemicals were seen in children living near petroleum refineries (67).

Aromatic amines are known to cause cancer at various sites including the bladder. In addition to the above-mentioned compounds, carcinogenicity to the human bladder has been proven for benzidine, 4-amino-biphynyl, and 2-naphthalamine (67). Aromatic amines can be generated as byproducts of petroleum refining and remain as contaminants in petroleum products. Some aromatic amines are also added to cutting oil and petroleum products (5).

21.7.6.3 Coal Dust and Fly Ash
Coal dust and fly ash are generated in power plants as a by-product of combustion. Coal dust and fly ash floating in the air can get into the lungs and cause respiratory difficulties. Persistent exposure to coke dust can cause pneumonitis and cancers of the urinary tract (2). It was well established that chimney sweeps in Britain developed scrotal cancer (7). Coke oven workers are often heavily exposed to polynuclear aromatic hydrocarbons and benzo(a) pyrene (8). Indeed, benzene and acetone-extracted samples of airborne particulate matter collected in two coke plants showed genotoxic agents such as polycyclic aromatic hydrocarbons, benzo(a)pyrene, dibenzo(a,h)anthracene, anthracene, and fluroanthracene. Coal dust and fly ash contain several heavy metals. Toxicity of some of the heavy metals is given next.

21.7.6.4 Lead
Lead poisoning can affect almost all organ systems. Acute exposure can cause nausea, vomiting, and death. Chronic exposure occurs by inhaling lead dust and lead oxide in an occupational setting. It can cause headache,

disturbance in thinking and cognitive function, disturbance in coordination, and peripheral neuropathy. Lead is an established animal and human carcinogen. Brain cancer mortality rates were greater in individuals exposed in an occupational setting than those not exposed to lead (**5,68**).

21.7.6.5 *Mercury*

Elemental mercury can be absorbed following vapor inhalation. The respiratory system is primarily affected. Pneumonitis, necrotizing bronchitis, pulmonary edema, and death can occur. With chronic exposure, nervous system changes predominate. Personality changes, hallucinations, headache, memory loss, altered sense of smell and taste, anorexia, and digestive system changes may occur. Carcinogenicity to animals and humans is not well-established (**5**).

21.7.6.6 *Arsenic*

Arsenic can be absorbed through the GI tract and can penetrate the intact skin. It can enter the body through inhalation. Acute exposure results in clinical symptoms as early as 30 minutes. Symptoms include burning lips, throat constriction, abdominal pain, muscle cramps, facial edema, bronchitis, chest pain, dehydration, and fluid and electrolyte disturbances. Inhalation of arsenic compounds is the route of exposure in an occupational setting. Arsenic is an established human and animal carcinogen. In humans, it causes sino-nasal cancer, skin carcinomas, bladder cancer, and pulmonary cancer. Thus far, there are no reports to suggest that it can cause cancer of the brain (**5**).

21.7.6.7 *Asbestos*

Asbestos is a known human carcinogen and the respiratory tract is the usual target organ. Asbestos exposure may cause autoimmune disorders and suppression of immune function resulting in increased infections. Fatigue and weight loss are common in patients with asbestosis. The primary types of asbestos-related cancers are mesothelioma of the pleura and peritoneum and broncogenic carcinoma. Some reports suggest an association between asbestos exposure and gastrointestinal or laryngeal malignancies (**2**). Exposure to asbestos occurs in an occupational setting by inhalation or ingestion of water containing asbestos particulates. Even though the lung is the primary target organ, asbestos is reported to cause cancer of the gastrointestinal tract, kidneys, pancreas, and brain. Epidemiological studies suggested that asbestos was a risk factor for brain cancer in workers exposed to asbestos. This is consistent with the incidence of brain cancer and mortality among asbestos insulation workers in the United States and Canada. A published case report showed the detection of asbestos in the brain tissue of an astrocytoma in a man who had a history of asbestos exposure for eight years. He was doing piping work in a shipyard (**66**).

21.7.6.8   Electric and Magnetic Field

Epidemiological studies suggest no association between electric and magnetic field (EMF) exposure and incidence of brain cancer in residential populations. However, meta-analysis in occupational settings indicated slightly higher risk for brain cancer in electrical workers. Some researchers have postulated that EMF may work in the promotion and progression of brain cancer. Among these populations, EMF exposure to organic solvents may play a significant role in the incidence of brain cancer. All the studies examined thus far report a very small increased risk of brain cancer (**69,70**).

21.7.7   Inadequate Industrial Hygiene Practices at Bloomfield Power Plant

As a technician, Mr. Delmick used Varsol to degrease the equipment. Some small parts were put into the Varsol tank or, if the parts are large, they were sprayed under pressure with Varsol. He was exposed to this varsol spray. There was very poor ventilation. Varsol used up to the middle of 1980 contained 25% benzene and the remainder is a mixture of hydrocarbons obtained from the petroleum distillate. In addition, Mr. Delmick was exposed to electrosol, which contained trichloroethane. These hydrocarbons have been established as animal and human carcinogens (**5**). Once it was recognized that benzene was a human carcinogen, recommendations were made for stringent industrial hygiene practices. In 1971, OSHA put a 10-ppm exposure limit on benzene and by 1976, OSHA and NIOSHA recommended a 1-ppm exposure of benzene. In 1987, OSHA set a limit of 1 ppm of benzene for an 8-hour day, time weighted average (TWA). OSHA also required medical surveillance for workers exposed to benzene, at specified intervals, and some companies have automated this data to monitor the health of their employees. The petroleum industry is well aware of the toxicity and carcinogenic potential of benzene other hydrocarbons and the consequences of exposure (**63,71**). One hundred years of experience with benzene and its toxicity made the federal government pass laws regulating benzene exposure by workers dealing or being exposed to benzene. The code of federal regulations became effective in December 1987. The 29 CFR. 1916. 1028 were published in *Federal Register* **52**:34460–34578, 1987. These regulations clearly state that the employer shall assure that no employee is exposed to an airborne concentration in excess of 1 ppm in an 8–hour TWA. There shall be a periodic medical surveillance program for those who are or who may be exposed to benzene. The medical examinations are to be performed by a qualified physician, and should include laboratory tests for blood cell count (**72**). No such recommendations by OSHA were followed at the power plant.

There was no proper protective equipment available to the workers. There was no proper ventilation at the plant where Mr. Delmick worked. There was fly ash all over and no data were collected to monitor the particulates the workers were inhaling. There is no evidence that data on heavy metals, arsenic, and asbestos present in the environment surrounding the workers was collected and monitored. There was no periodic data collected on the levels of EMF at the plant site. Even though management was aware of the chemicals present at the plant site, no MSDS were provided to the workers.

21.7.8   Development of Erick Delmick's Brain Cancer

Development of cancer is a two-step process. In animal models, it was clearly demonstrated that a carcinogen acts on a normal cell converting it to an initiated cell. This initiated cell lies dormant unless acted upon by a promoter. A promoter can be the same chemical or another agent, diet, or hormone. During this promotion phase, cancer develops and then during the progression stage, a full-blown tumor develops. It is recognized that there is a long latency period from the time a normal cell becomes an initiated cell and progresses to a tumor (**73**).

It is established that people in certain occupations such as electrical and petrochemical industries and farmers are at highest risk for brain cancer. The underlying agents in these groups of workers were shown to be their occupational exposure to chemicals and mineral oils that contain aliphatic and aromatic hydrocarbons. In the occupations with a high risk of inhalation and skin exposure of these hydrocarbons, there is increased incidence of brain cancer. The astrocytoma development increases with duration of employment. In the same occupational setting, the risk for brain cancer was elevated in workers who were considered to have no exposure to EMF. The inference is that these workers were exposed to solvents and a variety of chemicals other than EMF. A similar situation existed in workers in the petrochemical industry. The astrocytic tumors were elevated among subjects with production and maintenance jobs who had considerable exposure to organic chemicals (**74,75**).

Even though Mr. Delmick was exposed to asbestos, EMF, arsenic, lead, and other heavy metals, his tumor developed because of his chronic daily exposure to benzene and other hydrocarbons present in the degreasers that he used in the repair and maintenance of electrical equipment. He was exposed to these carcinogens early in his employment and the astrocytoma developed after a long latency period.

21.7.9 Conclusions

The following conclusions can be made with a reasonable degree of scientific certainty:

1. There was inadequate industrial hygiene at the Bloomfield Power Plant.
2. Periodic monitoring of occupational exposure of workers to toxins was not performed.
3. The management did not put in place periodic medical surveillance for those who are or who might be exposed to benzene and other toxins.
4. The medical examinations by a qualified physician, which include laboratory tests and blood cell counts, was not done.
5. Recommendations by OSHA were not followed at the power plant.
6. Mr. Delmick was exposed to asbestos, EMF, arsenic lead, and other heavy metals, which contributed to tumor development.
7. In addition, his tumor might have developed because of his chronic daily exposure to benzene and other hydrocarbons present in the degreasers used during the repair and maintenance of electrical equipment.
8. He was exposed to these carcinogens early in his employment and the astrocytoma developed after a long latency period.
9. The management at the Bloomfield Power Plant was solely responsible for the pain, suffering, and death of Mr. Delmick.

References

1. Wikipedia. Workers' compensation. http://en.wikipedia.org/wiki/Workers'_compensation.
2. Legal Information Institute. Workers' compensation: an overview. Cornell University Law School. http://topics.law.cornell.edu/wex/workers_compensation.
3. Expert Law. Pennsylvania workers' compensation benefits—An overview. http://www.expertlaw.com/library/comp_by_state/Pennsylvania.html.
4. Worker Compensation Law. http://worker-comp-law.com/.
5. Micromedix Health Care Service. Computer software for health professionals, 2001.
6. Ullrich, S.E. and Lyons, H.S. Mechanisms involved in the immunotoxicity induced by dermal application of JP-8 jet fuel. *Toxicol. Sci.* **58**:290–298, 2000.
7. Harris, D.T., Sakiestewa, D., Robledo, R.F., Young, R.S., and Witten, M. Effects of short-term JP-8 jet fuel exposure on cell mediated immunity. *Toxicol. Ind. Health* **16**:78–84, 2000.
8. Dudley, A.C., Peden-Adams, M.M., Eudaly, J., Pollen Z.R.S., and Keil, D.E. An aryl hydrocarbon receptor independent mechanism of JP-8 jet fuel immunotoxicity in An-responsive and ak-nonresponsive mice. *Toxicol. Sci.* **59**:251–259, 2001.
9. Ullrich, S.E. Dermal application of JP-8 jet fuel induces immune suppression. *Toxicol. Sci.* **52**:61–67, 1999.

10. Harris, D.T., Sakiestewa, D., Robledo, R.F., and Witten, M. Protection from JP-8 jet fuel induced immunotoxicity by administration of aerosolized substance P. *Toxicol. Ind. Health* **13**:571–588, 1997.
11. Harris, D.T., Sakiestewa, D., Robledo, R.F., and Witten, M. Short-term exposure to JP-8 jet fuel results in long-term immunotoxicity. *Toxicol. Ind. Health* **13**:559–570, 1997.
12. Harris, D.T., Sakiestewa, D., Robledo, R.F., and Witten, M. Immunotoxicological effects of JP-8 jet fuel exposure. *Toxicol. Ind. Health* **13**:43–55, 1997.
13. Rosenthal, G.J. and Snyder, C.A. Inhaled benzene reduces aspects of cell mediation tumor surveillance in mice. *Toxicol. Appl. Pharmacol.* **88**:35–43, 1987.
14. Rosenthal, G.J. and Snyder, C.A. Modulation of immune response to *Listeria monocytogenes* by benzene inhalation. *Toxicol. Appl. Pharmacol.* **80**:502–510, 1985.
15. Rosenthal, N.E. Multiple chemical sensitivity: lessons from seasonal affective disorder. *Toxicol. Ind. Health* **10**:623–632, 1994.
16. Anonymous. 29 CFR 1910, 1028. *Fed. Reg.* **52**:34460–34578, 198.
17. Di Maio,V.J. and Di Maio, D. *Forensic Pathology,*2nd ed. CRC Press, Boca Raton, FL, 2001.
18. Levine, B. *Principles of Forensic Toxicology.* AACC Press, Washington, DC. 1999.
19. Kaye, S. The collection and handling of blood alcohol specimens. *Am. J. Clin. Pathol.* **74**:743–746, 1980.
20. Heatly, M.K. The relationship between blood and urine alcohol concentrations at autopsy. *Med. Sci. Law* **29**:209–217, 1989.
21. Williams, R.H. and Leikin, J.B. Medicolegal issues and specimen collection for ethanol testing. *Lab. Med.* 530–537, 1999.
22. Chaturvedi, A.K., Smith, D.R., Soper, J.W., Confield, D.V., and Whinnery, J.F. Characteristics and toxicological processing of postmortem pilot specimens from fatal civil aviation accidents. Final Report. U.S. Department of Transportation. August 2002.
23. Sylvester, P.A., Wong, A.A.C.S., Warren, B.F., and Ranson, D.L. Unacceptably high site variability in postmortem blood alcohol analysis. *J. Clin. Pathol.* **51**:250–252, 1998.
24. Stowell, A.R. and Stowell, L.I. Estimation of blood alcohol concentrations after social drinking. *J. Forensic Sci.* **43**:14–21, 1998.
25. Lands, W.E.M. A review of alcohol clearance in humans. *Alcohol* **15**:147–160, 1998.
26. Winek, Jr., C.L., Winek C.L., and Whaba, W.W. The role of trauma in postmortem blood alcohol determination. *Forensic Sci. Int.* **71**:1–8, 1995.
27. Nine, J.S., Motaca, M., Virji, M.A., and Rao, K.N. Serum ethanol determination: Comparison of lactate and lactate dehydrogenase interference in three enzymatic assays. *J. Anal. Toxicol.* **19**:192–196, 1995.
28. Chang, L.W. (Ed.). *Toxicology of Metals.* CRC/Lewis Publishers, New York, 2000.
29. Occupational asthma: current perspective. www.agins.com/hew/resource/ocasthma.htm.
30. Calverley, A.E., Rees, D., Dowdeswell, R.J., Linnett, P.J., and Kielkowski, D. Platinum salt sensitivity in refinery workers: incidence and effects of smoking and exposure. *Occup. Environ. Med.* **52**:661–666, 1995.
31. Duenen, M., Rogiers, Ph., Van de Walle, C., Rochette, F., Demedts, M., and Nemery, B. Occupational asthma caused by palladium. *Eur. Respir. J.* **13**:213–216, 1999.

32. Merget, R., Reineke, M., Rueckmann, A., Bergman, E.M., and Schultze-Werninghaus, G. Nonspecific and specific bronchial responsiveness in occupational asthma caused by platinum salts after allergen avoidance. *Am. J. Respir. Crit. Care Med.* **150**:1146–1149, 1994.

33. Merget, R., Kulzer, R., Dierkes-Globisch, A., Breitstadt, R., Diplstat, A.G., Kniffka, A., Artelts, S., Koenig, H.P., Alt, F., Vomberg, R., Baur, X., and Schultze-Werninghaus, G., Exposure-effect relationship of platinum salt allergy in a catalyst production plant: Conclusions from a 5-year prospective cohort study. *J. Allergy Clin. Immunol.* **105**:364–370, 2000.

34. Merget, R., Schulte, A., Gehler, A., Breitstadt, R., Kulzer, R., Berndt, E.D., Baur, X., and Schultze-Werninghaus, G. Outcome of occupational asthma due to platinum salts after transfer to low-exposure area. *Inf. Arch. Occu. Environ. Health* **72**:33–39, 1999.

35. Merget, R., Caspari, C., Dierkes-Globisch, A., Kulzer, R., Breitstadt, R., Kniffka, A., Degens, P., and Schultze-Werninghaus, G. Effectiveness of a medical surveillance program for the prevention of occupational asthma caused by platinum salts: a nested case control study. *J. Allergy Clin. Immunol.* **107**:707–712, 2001.

36. Mapp, C., Boschetto, P., Miotto, D., DeRosa, E., and Fabric, L. Mechanisms of occupational asthma. *Am. Col. Allergy Asthma Immunol.* **83**:645–666, 1999.

37. Cantarell, M.C., Fort, J., Camps, J., Sans, M., Piera, L., and Rodamilans, M. Acute intoxication due to topical application of diethylene glycol. *Ann. Int. Med.* **106**:478–479, 1987.

38. Lynch, K.M. Diethylene glycol poisoning. *South. Med. J.* **31**:134–137, 1938.

39. Lenk, W., Lohr, D., and Sonnenbichler, J. Pharmacokinetics and biotransformation of diethylene glycol and ethylene glycol in rats. *Xenobiotica* **19**:961–979, 1989.

40. Mathews, J.M., Parker, M.K., and Matthews, H.B. Metabolism and disposition of diethylene glycol in rat and dog. *Drug Metab. Dispos.* **19**:1066–1070, 1991.

41. Okuonghae, H.O., Ighogboja, I.S., Lawson, J.O., and Nwaana, J.C. Diethylene glycol poisoning in Nigerian children. *Ann. Trop. Paediatr.* **12**:235–238, 1992.

42. Hanif, M., Mobarak, M.R., Ronan, A., Rahman, D., Donovan, J.J., and Bennish, M.L. Fatal renal failure by diethylene glycol in paracetamol elixir: the Bangladesh experience. *BMJ* **311**: 88–91, 1995.

43. Woolf, A.D. The Haitian diethylene glycol poisoning tragedy: A dark wood revisited. *JAMA* **279**:1215–1216, 1998.

44. Hasbani, M.J., Sansing, L.H., Perrono, J., Asbury, A.K., and Bird, S.J. Encephalopathy and peripheral neuropathy following diethylene glycol ingestion. *Neurology* **64**:1273–1275, 2005.

45. Karch, S.B. *Pathology of Drug Abuse.* CRC Press, Boca Raton, FL, 2002.

46. Baselt, R.C. and Cravey, R.H. *Disposition of Toxic Drugs Chemicals in Man.* Chemical Toxicology Institute, Foster City, CA, 1995.

47. Metal finishing. www.electronicssouth.com/index.cfm.

48. Derelanko, M.J. Carcinogenesis. In: *Handbook of Toxicology.* M.J. Derelanko and M.A. Hallanger, Eds. CRC Press, Boca Raton, FL, 1995, 357–358.

49. Bonner, H. The blood and the lymphoid organs. In: *Pathology.* E. Rubin and J.L. Farber, Eds. J.B. Lippincott Co., Philadelphia, PA, 1988, 1014–1117.

50. Lymphoma Information Network. Hodgkin's lymphoma (Hodgkin's disease). www.lymphomainfo.net/hodgkins.

51. MedicineNet. Non-Hodgkin's lymphoma. www.medicinenet.com/non-hodg-kins_lymphomas.
52. Norseth, T. The carcinogenicity of chromium. *Environ. Health Perspect.* **40**:121–130, 1981.
53. Chromium hexavalent salts. Micromedix Health Care series.
54. Klein, C.B. Carcinogenicity and genotoxicity of chromium. In: *Toxicology of Metals.* L.W. Chang, Ed. CRC/ Lewis Publishers, New York, 1996, 205–219.
55. Mancuso, T.F. Chromium as an industrial carcinogen: part I. *Am. J. Ind. Med.* **31**:129–139, 1997.
56. Ziegler, V. and Ziegler, B. Experimentally induced malignant lymphoma due to chronic antigen stimulation. *Contact Derm.* **30**:77–79, 1994.
57. Bick, R.L., Girardi, T.V., Lack, W.J., Costa, M., and Titelbaum, D. Hodgkin's disease in association with hexavalent chromium exposure. *Int. J. Hematol.* **64**:257–262, 1996.
58. Ming, W. and Ping, W. Occupational risk factors for selected cancers. *Am. J. Public Health* **94**:1078–1080, 2004.
59. Briggs, N.C., Levine, R.S., Hall, I.H., Cosby, O., Brann, E.A., and Hennekens, C.H. Occupational risk factors for selected cancers among African American and White men in the United States. *Am. J. Public Health* **93**:1748–1752, 2003.
60. Brinton, H.P., Fraser, E.S., and Koven, A.L. Morbidity and mortality experience among chromate workers. *Public Health Rep.* **67**:835–847, 1952.
61. Pan, S.Y., Ugnat, A.M., and Mao, Y. Occupational risk factors for brain cancer in Canada. *J. Occup. Environ. Med.* **47**:704–717, 2005.
62. Cotran, R.S., Kumar, V., and Robbins, S.L. *Robbins Pathologic Basis of Disease*, 5th ed. W. B. Saunders, Philadelphia, PA, 1994, 1342–1343.
63. Raab, G.K. and Wong, O. Leukemia mortality by cell type in petroleum workers with potential exposure to benzene. *Environ. Health Perspect.* **104**:1381–1392, 1996.
64. Panstenback, D.J., Bass, R.D., and Price, P. Benzene toxicity and risk assessment, 1972–1992. Implications for future regulations. *Environ. Health Perspect.* **101** (suppl. 6):177–200, 1993.
65. Snyder, R. and Heldi, C.C. An overview of benzene metabolism. *Environ. Health Perspect.* **104** (suppl.6): 1165–1171, 1996.
66. Boffetta, P., Jowenkova, N., and Gustavson, P. Cancer risk from occupational and environmental exposure to polycyclic aromatic hydrocarbons. *Cancer Causes Control* **8**:444–474, 1997.
67. Arnold, J.P., Kubiak, R., Belowski, J., Belegand, J., and Sezezekilk, J. Detection of benzo(a)pyrene-DNA adducts in leukocytes of coke oven workers. *Pathol. Biol.* **48**:548–553, 2000.
68. Wijangaarden, E.V. and Dosemeel, M. Brain cancer mortality and potential occupational exposure to lead. Findings from the national longitudinal mortality study. 1979–1989. *Intl. J. Cancer* **119**:1136–1144, 2006.
69. Editorial. Occupational exposure to magnetic fields and brain cancer. *Occup. Environ. Med.* **58**:617–618, 2001.
70. Kheifets, L. I. Electric and magnetic field exposure and brain cancer: a review. *Bioelectromagnetics Suppl.* **5**:5120–5131, 2001.
71. Mehlman, M.A. Benzene health effects. Unanswered questions still not addressed. *Am. J. Ind. Med.* **20**:707–711, 1991.
72. Anonymous. 29CFR. 1910,1028. *Fed. Reg.* **52**:34460–34578, 1987.

73. Derelanko, M.J. Carcinogenesis. In: *Handbook of Toxicology.* M.J. Derelanko and M.A. Hallanger, Eds. CRC Press, Boca Raton, FL, 1995, 357–360.
74. Thomas, T.L., Stolley, P.D., Stemnagen, A., Fontham, E.T., Bleecker, M.L., Stewart, P.A., and Hoover, R.N. Brain tumor mortality risk among men with electrical and electronics jobs: case control study. *J. Natl. Cancer Inst.* **79**:233–238, 1987.
75. Thomas, T.L., Stewart, P.A., Stemhagen, A., Correa, P., Norman, S.A., Bleecker, M.L., and Hoover, R.N. Risk of astrocytic brain tumors associated with occupational chemical exposure. A case control study. *Scand. J. Work Environ. Health* **13**:417–423, 1987.

Index

For Product Safety Concerns and Information please contact our EU
representative GPSR@taylorandfrancis.com
Taylor & Francis Verlag GmbH, Kaufingerstraße 24, 80331 München, Germany